Practical Human Behaviour Change
for the Health and Welfare of Animals

Practical Human Behaviour Change for the Health and Welfare of Animals

Bronwen Williams RMN, PGCHE, MSc

WILEY Blackwell

Registered Offices
John Wiley & Sons, Inc., 111 River Street, Hoboken, NJ 07030, USA
John Wiley & Sons Ltd, The Atrium, Southern Gate, Chichester, West Sussex, PO19 8SQ, UK

For details of our global editorial offices, customer services, and more information about Wiley products visit us at www.wiley.com.

Wiley also publishes its books in a variety of electronic formats and by print-on-demand. Some content that appears in standard print versions of this book may not be available in other formats.

Library of Congress Cataloging-in-Publication Data
Names: Williams, Bronwen, 1964– author.
Title: Practical Human Behaviour Change for the Health and Welfare of Animals /
     by Bronwen Williams.
Description: Hoboken, NJ : John Wiley & Sons Ltd, 2024. | Includes
     bibliographical references and index.
Identifiers: LCCN 2023028997 (print) | LCCN 2023028998 (ebook) | ISBN
     9781394178858 (paperback) | ISBN 9781394178865 (adobe pdf) | ISBN
     9781394178872 (epub) | ISBN 9781394178889 (ebook)
Subjects: LCSH: Animal specialists–Psychology. | Volunteer workers in
     animal shelters–Psychology | Animal welfare–Psychological aspects |
     Motivational interviewing. | Behavior modification. | Human-animal
     relationships.
Classification: LCC SF80 .W55 2024 (print) | LCC SF80 (ebook) | DDC
     636.08/32019–dc23/eng/20231214
LC record available at https://lccn.loc.gov/2023028997
LC ebook record available at https://lccn.loc.gov/2023028998

Cover Design: Wiley
Cover Images: © mgstudyo/Getty Images, © AzmanL /Getty Images

Set in 9.5/12.5pt STIXTwoText by Straive, Pondicherry, India

Contents

Foreword

The skills covered in this book – which were taught to me by the author – have had the single biggest impact of anything I have learned in over two decades working in animal welfare.

I have lost count of the number of owners I have spoken to about their horses through the roles I have held at World Horse Welfare over the past 20 years. I am office-based, so my conversations have largely taken place over the phone, and these skills have proven invaluable in that context. Many of my colleagues, who have undertaken the same training, speak face to face with a huge variety of horse owners and other individuals on a daily basis. I have the privilege of a rare insight into the work they do, the challenges they face and the way in which so many of them have embedded these skills into that work in order to help horses – and their owners – as effectively as possible.

I first met Bronwen back in 2016 when she gave a fascinating presentation on animal hoarding behaviour to some of the World Horse Welfare team. Bronwen has a great depth of knowledge and experience to draw on: she is a mental health nurse with 42 years' experience working in the NHS, volunteered in equine welfare for 30 years and has been a trainer of motivational interviewing for 22 years. I was privileged to be given the opportunity to complete a motivational interviewing course in 2019, delivered by Bronwen, which was primarily aimed at World Horse Welfare's team of field officers. This approach has since become embedded within the organisation, as a number of colleagues across various roles and departments have been trained over the past few years, with more to come in future. I could not have predicted the profound impact that course would have on me and the way I communicate, not just with owners but with colleagues, friends, family and even with strangers. More recently, I have been fortunate to co-train with Bronwen, delivering this training to others in the animal welfare world, and in turn have continued benefitting from her considerable knowledge. Bronwen would be the first to say that the skills covered in this book are no magic solution. They will not suit everyone, nor will they work in every situation.

However, I have been amazed at the range of circumstances in which my colleagues and I have successfully used various different elements, and how it has helped to enable purposeful conversations in very difficult situations. The skills can be challenging to learn, and it takes work to embed them into practice, but for me and many of my colleagues, the outcomes have justified every ounce of effort put in.

Many animal health and welfare workers face the same regular frustrations. They encounter particular scenarios unfolding time and again with different people. They see owners repeating certain undesirable behaviours, despite the worker's best interventions. Workers are sometimes desperate to share critical information but find their audience unwilling to receive it, or they might even have thrown their hands up in despair, feeling that, however hard they try, nothing they do makes a difference. Whilst we can all absorb this if it only happens occasionally, it can quickly build up and start to have a noticeable impact on the individual: the risk of compassion fatigue and burnout in the animal welfare world is widely recognised. However, I hope that this book will provide some insight into how you can build on your own significant, existing knowledge and experience by giving you fresh ways to approach these long-standing difficulties. I have witnessed how these skills have not only helped to resolve welfare situations more quickly and effectively but also have been used peer to peer to facilitate better outcomes and allow constructive reflection on – and indeed, preparation for – difficult conversations and situations, therefore helping to mitigate some of this risk.

One of my colleagues remarked that, thanks to this training, she now has the ability to be able to handle any scenario that comes her way. Whilst she acknowledges that she won't always have the right answer, she now has the skills to help people and to have a conversation about absolutely anything, and I know she is not alone in feeling that way. I hope this book will give you the same confidence.

Sam Chubbock
Head of UK Support, World Horse Welfare

Preface

Introduction to the Contents and How They Might Be Used to Develop Your Skills

This book is designed to support anyone whose main element of their work is animal health, care, or welfare as well as those who come across animal welfare issues as part of their wider roles. You may need animal owners to make changes for the welfare of their animals, and perhaps for their own good and that of others or even communities and the environment.

It is designed to be accessible and suitable for all types of workers, including those employed in animal health, care, welfare, veterinary work, charities, rescues or volunteering, those having to enforce animal welfare legislation, and those in associated agencies who come across animal welfare cases such as environmental health, trading standards, and housing workers.

For all of us, changing behaviour is difficult. When we work with others, especially in animal health and welfare, we desperately need people to change their behaviours for the well-being of animals. But behaviour change is not easy for anyone, and few people respond well to being told what to do and that they need to make changes.

No book can take the place of learning face-to-face, especially with the skills required for supporting behaviour change, including one of the main interventions described in this book, motivational interviewing (MI). However, it is hoped that working through the chapters will help the reader think about themselves as well as others, and about how we all make changes and then to consider what skills work and what don't and how we can build on our existing abilities to support others to make changes.

This book is the culmination of several decades of teaching the intervention called MI to health and social care staff and more recently, to animal welfare workers. It has come out of the author's interest in how human mental health can be affected, for good or for ill, by animal ownership or responsibility for animals.

The author is a mental health nurse who has worked clinically in the NHS for many decades as well as an educator both in the NHS and in higher education and as an independent trainer for animal welfare agencies. She also volunteered as an equine welfare worker for over 30 years and used the techniques she teaches in that work.

MI was initially developed as an intervention for those with substance misuse problems and its use has moved into a number of other human health areas such as working with those with other addictive behaviours (e.g. gambling) and within smoking cessation programmes. It hadn't been recognised as an intervention that can transfer across to supporting those who need, or are required, to make changes in their behaviour for the well-being, welfare, and health of animals. As a mental health nurse trained in MI and then delivering training to mental health colleagues, the author found herself automatically using MI approaches and skills when undertaking equine volunteer work over three decades. Conversations about MI occurred with other equine welfare workers and the organisations that they worked for. Now, the MI training courses have been adapted and developed specifically for those who work with animal owners and carers. This book is based on, and supports, those courses. Much of the content of this book has come about through the experiences of teaching MI to a wide range of people, listening to how they go on to use it in their own practice, and also the author's own human clinical work and animal welfare experience. Many of the examples given in this book are from those who have successfully transferred the ideas and skills to their own work.

Many people have helped the author along this road, not least as her co-trainers over the years, especially Keith Noble, Beth Stranks, and Kelly Skinner, with whom many conversations have helped form or develop the ideas here and who are mentioned specifically in places in the book. Many people from the international equine charity World Horse Welfare have shared their experiences of learning and using MI in their welfare work and supported the development of MI in the animal welfare arena. Specifically, Sam Chubbock, who really 'gets it' and has been a co-trainer as well as one of the author's writing buddies. Also, Claire Gordon who first identified that the author's ideas could be used within World Horse Welfare; and Tony Tyler and Roly Owers who supported this work and have been so enthusiastic about its use in the organisation. Finally, a friend, Ian Glass whose greatest support was just listening when it was most needed.

How to Develop the Skills Described in This Book

Throughout the book, you will find suggestions of how you might take elements, techniques, or approaches and practice them. Try finding willing friends, family, and colleagues to help you and who will allow you to practice with them. Almost everyone likes to talk about what they might change in their lives, especially their own health behaviour changes. This means that we can usually find people who will help us on our journey of learning about how to support others to make changes. But bear in mind that it can be very hard to practice with those closest to us. Often, we have a vested interest in a possible change, so sometimes family members especially, and others we are close to, can be more challenging for us personally than some of those we might come in contact with at work or in our other roles.

The ideas and approaches described in this book are not designed to manipulate people into doing what we want, so please undertake any practice openly and for the right reasons. That said, when we ask others for support when we are learning new techniques, very few will say no. I have had a few people report back after practicing some of the skills on their partners that it was not easy, even when the partner had agreed to help them practice. One student who decided to try the skills on their husband, but without telling him, had the response, 'Why are you being weird?' Although it was funny and made her colleagues in the training group laugh when she shared it, this demonstrates that people, especially those who know us well, will pick up very quickly that we are being 'different'.

Therefore, look for opportunities to practice with people, be prepared to ask them for help in supporting you in using new approaches. People can be very generous in their time and help, so use it. I suggest you look for those who may aid you to practice the techniques in the early stages, who will work with you and are not as complex as some of your other work.

Many of us come to behaviour change and MI courses, literature, or a book like this looking for the key, or the magic wand, to resolving the most difficult cases or owners that we have. I suggest that instead, we start with those who will be slightly easier for us. I liken this approach to that of learning to drive. When we start out on our first driving lessons, we usually have a suitable smaller, lower-powered car (some of us may have started out on ancient tractors). We wouldn't put a learner driver in a high-powered sports car. We give them a chance to learn with something that isn't so tricky and is more forgiving to errors and adjustments. Therefore, I suggest you find people to practice with or to try out the skills with who are the least complex of your clients, owners, or friends and family. Learn with a Ford Fiesta or an Opal Corsa, not a Ferrari!

Get feedback from anyone you can find to practice with. Many of the suggested exercises in the book can be used with willing friends, family, and colleagues. But our greatest feedback can be from our clients and owners, so ask their views about what helped, what didn't, and what they think we might have done differently. When asked, clients can be very generous with their help. Also, be realistic about what you can learn in a short period of time, and give yourself opportunities to practice, refine your skills and adapt the new ideas and techniques into your own particular style of working.

It can be, at the very least, disheartening and frustrating to feel that we are working with people who won't or don't do what we recommend or advise. Over time, this can wear any one of us down and affect how we feel about our role and its worth. The good news is that those who I have taught MI to over the decades, often report that they enjoy their work more, it is less stressful, and that they experience more job satisfaction and less friction with their clients and other colleagues.

Learning to use different methods to support others to make behaviour changes is in itself a behaviour change for us. Therefore, we need to use with ourselves the same approaches and attitudes described in this book when we endeavour to make changes and learn new skills. Everything takes practice, effort and thought and that is very much the case when changing our approaches and the ways that we work with others. Be kind and compassionate to yourself, be prepared to have a go, try out new ideas, and techniques and reflect when they work and when they don't work so well. Be curious, and prepared for the unexpected. Find a little time to reflect on your practice. Perhaps even write down some notes or use a journal. As professionals, we all need to reflect on our practice. But, be balanced in your reflections, think about what skills you do already have, and how the ideas offered here in this book add to and build on those skills.

Remember, change isn't easy for anyone. It takes time and effort, and we need to make mistakes in order to perfect our approaches and to develop. Working through the ideas, skills, and techniques in this book is no different.

How to Use This Book

The book is designed for you to move through the chapters, but with reminders of ideas and skills that were mentioned earlier in the book. Especially in the chapters that describe and outline particular techniques, it will be useful to return to them perhaps a number of times to refresh yourself with some of the underpinning ideas discussed earlier and linked to in that particular chapter.

One chapter that it is suggested you revisit most frequently is the active listening chapter, as this underpins everything else. Without the skills outlined in that chapter, helping others to change their behaviours is very unlikely to be successful. In our courses, we know that if we don't include some active listening practice on day one, the rest of the course doesn't go so well. We still do this with experienced human health clinicians, including mental health nurses, psychologists, and social workers who all know about active listening and usually have high levels of skill in this.

At the start of this introductory chapter, I said that this book doesn't take the place of face-to-face training and learning but is designed to be as close to that as possible. Therefore, the moving backwards and forwards through the chapters allows you to build up layers of learning as you go. It has been written holding the reader in mind throughout and thinking of how the ideas can be best put across to help you and your clients get the best from your work.

Remember, if you are reading this book, it is very likely that you already have many skills and methods that work. Don't forget the skills that you do have and what you get right. Although learning and adapting to some of the ideas and skills may not always be easy, they will compliment your existing skills, rather than learning a whole new way of being with people. Think of it as a way of honing your approaches. Be confident in what you already do and what already works, and hopefully, this book will assist you to get different outcomes with people that will benefit them, you and most of all, their animals.

Are you now ready to make some changes to how you work?

About the Companion Website

Practical Human Behaviour Change for the Health and Welfare of Animals is accompanied by a companion website:

www.wiley.com/go/williams/human

The website includes:

- Templates

1

Understanding What Lies Behind Behaviours

1.1 Introduction

This chapter outlines some ideas that can help us understand why people may behave as they do. One idea, the *frame of reference*, can help explain and so aid our understanding about why people develop views, attitudes and underpinning beliefs and values that drive behaviours. Understanding someone's perspective, or frame of reference, and how their situation came about, can significantly improve our knowledge of them and their world, thus aiding us to engage and help them. Through understanding, but not necessarily agreeing with or condoning someone's behaviour, we can help them feel listened to without judgment. Enabling someone to talk about how they arrived at their current situation allows us, and often the owners themselves, to more fully understand their backstory.

1.2 Behaviour Change Is Difficult

We have all made behaviour changes throughout our lives. Some of these changes have worked, and we have stuck with them. Some haven't, and we gave up and returned to old behaviours. Perhaps we have stopped, started, stopped, and then again restarted some behaviours. Thinking about the behaviours we have changed, those that were successful, and those that didn't work out, or at least not at first attempt, gives clues about how change is neither simple nor straightforward for anyone. This includes changes that people need to make for the well-being of their animals. People arrive in their current situation due to particular and unique experiences. People's behaviours, including those that may need to change, will be underpinned by beliefs, values and experiences.

Practical Human Behaviour Change for the Health and Welfare of Animals, First Edition. Bronwen Williams.

Box 1.1   Exercise

You might take a couple of minutes to think about behaviour changes you have made over time, even in your lifetime. Which ones stuck? Which didn't? With what you know now, what would you do differently?

Beliefs, values, and traditions underpin much of how humans behave and often influence how they relate to animals in their lives. Understanding these and how they underpin behaviours, especially if people hold different values and views to ours, will be essential to supporting behaviour change for animal health and welfare. Owners, and others', experiences are going to be important to help us understand them and to appreciate how they got to their current circumstances. Someone's backstory is key: how they came to be where they are when we encounter them. Often, this backstory is much more complex, interesting, or unusual than we could ever imagine. We just need to ask in the right way and, more importantly, listen in the right way, to get an understanding of this backstory.

Box 1.2   Example – A Backstory

An example of this is a very moving backstory told by my colleague Jan about her neighbour, Mary. Mary could be somewhat irritating for others living in their close community. She often did things that appeared thoughtless to others, although she was recognised as being generally well meaning. Those living nearby, including Jan, were very amused by Mary's anger when her plants were suddenly eaten by wildlife. Then, one day, Jan had the presence of mind to ask Mary why these particular plants were so important to her. Out came a backstory that was very unexpected, detailed, and so personal that the finer points were never shared with others, including me. As soon as Jan understood Mary's reasons, why these plants were so important, she felt very differently towards her. Instead of being frustrated and joining in with other neighbours who found Mary's upset funny, Jan now understood Mary's position. She could empathise greatly with her, and their relationship deepened and was much more tolerant from both sides. One simple enquiry – stopping to ask the reason why something was important, getting the individual's backstory – and everything changed.

In the world of human psychological work, seeing a situation or an issue from a completely different perspective is known as a 'cognitive reframe'. Those who need to change their behaviour to improve the well-being of their animals often need to undertake a cognitive reframe or experience a change of perspective. I suggest that this also needs a cognitive reframe from others, including us as workers. We need to have professional curiosity, put our default perceptions to one side, and attempt to find out why something is happening to understand the other person's experience.

Box 1.3   Example – A Paradigm Shift

Stephen Covey, in his book *The 7 Habits of Highly Effective People*, tells a story of when he was on a train on a Sunday morning. All was peaceful until a man and his out-of-control children entered the carriage. While the kids ran riot, disturbing everyone's peace and quiet, the father seemed totally unaware and unbothered, much to the irritation of the other passengers. Eventually, Stephen Covey spoke to the man, drawing his attention to the way his children were behaving. The man then roused himself and apologised and said quietly that his wife, the childrens' mother, had just died in the hospital, and that he and the kids didn't know how to handle it. In that moment, Stephen Covey's whole perspective changed and his concern became focused on the bereaved family, what he calls a 'paradigm shift' – when a person sees a situation in a completely different way.

Whatever title we give this – 'paradigm shift', 'a cognitive reframe', or 'understanding the person's backstory' – whenever we can do it, it makes a huge difference to the quality of our engagement with someone and how we can work with them. It allows us to be more patient, understanding, and empathic. We don't have to agree with what they think or do, but we can get alongside them and be more effective. It can also mean that the work and any interactions can be easier for us as workers. Understanding and having empathy is hard but it is a lot easier than being the recipient of anger, frustration, and general annoyance from the person we are trying to work with.

A welfare colleague I was teaching described a response from an owner when they were called out to a welfare report, and which perhaps demonstrated a different and unexpected view. The owner, whose animals had no welfare issues, said, 'It's good, isn't it that someone cares enough about animals that they ask for their welfare to be checked?' What a great example of a very different view of the world!

We all have our own perspective or lens through which we see the world, and this is what we will look at in this chapter, along with what may support the development of our perspectives.

Box 1.4 Exercise

Take a couple of minutes to think about the cases in animal health, care, or welfare you have seen over your time working or volunteering in this field. Think about a couple of specific cases in which owners of animals had very different views, beliefs, or values from you and from the organisation you work for. They may have been small things or very big differences. Which ones come to your mind right now? How did you manage these? What impact did these differences have on your working relationship with those individual/s?

1.3 Frame of Reference

Where do people's beliefs and traditions originate from, whether these are general or specifically about animals? A model called the 'frame of reference', first coined by Schiff and Schiff (1975), suggests that we all have a complex set of assumptions and attitudes which allow individuals to assess and build meaning which creates a unique view of the world. This underpins how we see ourselves and everything else in the world. It gives us a 'filter on reality' or a lens through which we see things. The old adage of someone being a 'glass half-full or glass half-empty' type of person may be an example of a basic view on the world. If you are a glass half-full person, you tend to see the best in a situation, life and people, and a glass half-empty view of the world would be more pessimistic about life events and situations.

There is a saying about seeing things 'through rose-tinted glasses'; when one has a tendency to see situations in a positively biased way or by putting a warm and comfortable gloss on issues. The reality is that we all see the world, ourselves, and others in it through our own 'tinted glasses', but rather than being of one hue (rose coloured or otherwise), the world is viewed with very complex layers to our 'glasses'.

Depending on our beliefs, views, and current emotions as well as our backgrounds and experiences, our 'tinted glasses' or frame of reference will cause us to interpret reality, situations, and other people in a unique way. Our frame of reference may therefore be very different to other people's views, or interpretations of a very similar experience, issue, or event. Even those with whom we are closest – family, siblings, partners, spouses, friends, and colleagues – may interpret, experience and respond to something very differently from us.

This unique, complex lens on the world, our frame of reference, will affect how we make judgements, how we understand the world, ourselves and other people. It will impact how we view animals including those we own and those belonging to others. It also affects how we act or behave.

This frame of reference is developed by many things. The diagram below shows experiences, events, and individual traits that build an individual frame of reference or colours the lenses in our glasses through which we look at the world.

FRAME OF REFERENCE

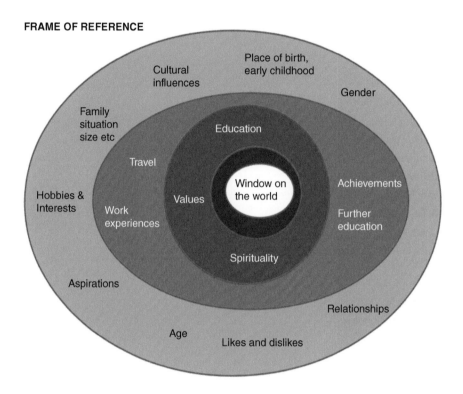

Box 1.5   Exercise Part 1

Spend a little time, if you would like to, thinking about your life experiences and what may have influenced you to see the world as you do, your frame of reference. You might want to make some brief notes in the form below if that is useful.
Next, consider if any of these factors from the frame of reference impact your view of animals? Has anything influenced you to do the work that you do with animals? Make a few notes in the last column against each of the areas

Some factors that may influence our view or frame of reference of the world	Notes about your own experience that may impact how you see the world	Notes about your own experience that may impact how you view animals
Inner circle		
Values		
Spirituality		
School / education		
Middle circle		
Further education		
Travel		
Work experiences		
Achievements		
Outer circle		
Family situation, size, etc.		
Relationships and friendships		
Gender		
Place of birth and Early childhood		
Age		
Aspirations		
Hobbies and interests		
Likes and dislikes		
Cultural influences		

Box 1.6   Exercise Part 2

What do you make of this exercise?

What stands out when you look at or think about your answers or notes in each area?

How might these be different from those of your closest friend, your partner or spouse, or even a sibling?

How do these experiences impact the way you act and behave in the world and the decisions and judgements that you make?

Box 1.7   Exercise Part 3

Now reflect on your beliefs, values, and attitudes towards animals and animal ownership (those you own and those others keep). Think about your beliefs and attitudes towards how animals should be fed, how they should be kept, and how they are used to work for humans or for food and other products. Lastly, think about your beliefs, values, and attitudes regarding the death of animals. Do you have views on euthanasia? Where do these beliefs and attitudes about euthanasia come from? Have these changed over time – if so, what influenced the changes?

1.4   Humans' Frame of Reference and How They See Animals

Each of us hold beliefs and values about animals and yours may have influenced your decision to work in animal health, care, or welfare. Your behaviour will be underpinned by a very individual and unique frame of reference, or view of the world. Many experiences and events, such as the areas outlined in the frame of reference, will affect how humans relate to and interact with animals (Dodman et al. 2018).

Let's look at each of those areas from the frame of reference again in a bit more detail and about how this might be for people who own animals.

1.4.1   Inner Circle of the Frame of Reference

Let's start with the inner circle. Values, spirituality, and education, all of which can develop very early on in life, can be very personal but evolve due to our experiences and the impact of other people upon us.

Values: Our values often come right from our earliest experiences in life. Whether or not life was good when we were children, helps form our values. People who were influential when we were young will significantly impact on our values about, and views of, animals. We all take on the values of those most important to us – our families; our communities; our spiritual, cultural, and religious experiences. Values may be re-evaluated and adjusted in adolescence and again in adulthood. Sometimes, as Serpell (2004) discusses, values and beliefs about animals can be held over many generations, even after they are no longer relevant or useful. As humans, we can therefore inherit some or even most of our values about animals that may have come from many generations before. These may be outdated and no longer appropriate, yet difficult to let go of as they form part of our history, identity, and feelings of connection and belonging.

In animal health and care work, when we need people to change their behaviours, it is important to explore, understand, and appreciate the beliefs and values that underpin their actions and decisions, or their lack thereof. This is the same no matter which country or continent we live and work in.

Spirituality: Spiritual perspectives on life and on animals may be formal and come from religions and cultures, or they may be personal, formulated by our thinking and own life experiences.

School/Education: Early education will probably lay the foundation for how we are able to access and develop in further and higher education. Animals and our relationships with them, in our early formative education may develop our views. Animals do tend to appear in stories and tales, modern and old. For example, *The Bible* has animals in it. Fairy tales have many animals, often as central characters, and many to be afraid of. Some schools have pets or some farmed animals such as chickens, to allow students to look after them and appreciate where food may come from.

1.4.2 Middle Circle of the Frame of Reference

Further Education: For many people, this may be minimal, or something that they did not experience at all. Further education usually means mixing with, often living among, people who may not have come from the same or even similar backgrounds as us. This allows us to widen our experiences of the world, sometimes through hearing other people's experiences or sharing our day to day lives with them. Further education teaches us to be more analytical, more critical, to question, and to change the ways in which we think and reason.

Serpell (2004) mentions that scientific developments and research can change how humans see animals. However, people need support through education and perhaps further education in order to become critical thinkers, and to take on what evidence scientific information presents, especially if it is completely different or at odds with how they have been brought up and to what they have been practicing for many years.

Travel: The ability to travel may be very limited in some of the communities you might work with, and for others, travelling experience may be much more extensive. Some people may not have had opportunities to be exposed to alternative ways of living, thinking, and working with or keeping or interacting with animals.

Work Experiences: Animals may feature in people's work lives in a variety of ways including farming, the leisure and tourism industry, pet and companion animal industries, conservation and wildlife, animal welfare, transportation, environmental and trading standards, pharmaceutical and other testing, butchery, food and other manufacturing, assistance animals, and working animals such as dogs and horses in the police and armed forces.

Cultures within work settings may impact upon an individual's frame of reference. People may hold particular views about, or attitudes towards, the animals they work with. These can be very different to how they view those they may have at home, such as companion animals. Work environments may mean that people have prolonged exposure to particular ways of treating animals, that then become the norm for them.

Achievements: What we have achieved, or aspire to achieve, can affect how we view ourselves and others, and the world as a whole, including the animals within it. For some, competing against others may be a way of aiming for or obtaining achievements. For some, activities such as breeding and showing animals can bring a sense of achievement. This may lead to welfare issues if the individual puts more value on the achievement rather than animal welfare. This can be seen in the breeding and animal showing world, when breeding is done in the pursuit of producing the winning animal, the one who will be held as high value by others or who may make or reinstate the breeder's reputation and social standing. This type of breeding for achievement, described as 'chasing the one' (Williams et al. 2020) can result in animals who do not meet the required standards being discarded as 'waste' products.

1.4.3 The Outer Circle of the Frame of Reference

The Family Situation / Size: The position a person is born into within a family, the eldest or youngest for example, may affect how they see the world and their place in it. The need to secure an income and resources for the family may be a key part of someone's life, especially for men in many cultures. A sense of responsibility for siblings or other family members or gender expectations and roles within a family will influence an individual's frame of reference. We can inherit our family's behaviours and beliefs about animals, but the unique experiences for each of us due to our place in our family and its dynamics can create differences in frames of reference even between siblings. Added to this, when animals are part of a family situation, whether as companion animals, farmed, hunted or as working animals, this will have an impact on how they are viewed and treated.

Gender: Our gender, and what it means to us – how we were treated as a child and growing up – may influence how we view the world. An example of this was an owner of a number of animals who came in contact with animal welfare workers. She had married young, had been expected to have children and did so, having a number in quick succession. This owner didn't want her animals rehomed as she was worried that the female animals would be used for breeding by those in her culture. This very personal experience led her to not want a similar life for her animals.

Relationships and Friendships: Relationships and friendships help form our frame of reference. Experiences with fellow humans can drive how people choose to keep or how they treat their animals. Peer pressure and requirements to fit in with a group or community can influence how we see the world. This may encourage people to obtain and keep animals similar to those which are owned by friends to enable them to be accepted into a group. This can happen with reptile keeping, for example. Other examples may be young men who obtain horses or ponies when they are living in urban areas without the appropriate environments for equines. Other people may choose to keep particular breeds of dogs which fit with an image that their group has and which they want to portray to others.

Groups that support people with young animals can have a significantly positive impact on the treatment and management of animals by new owners. An example of this is puppy training courses. More problematic may be groups of young adolescents who influence each other to seek out and torment or harm animals. An individual might not have done this on their own but may take part when they are part of a social group and experience peer pressure.

Place of Birth and Early Childhood: Birth and how children are raised, especially in the very early years, will have a huge impact on their frame of reference. Attachments with primary caregivers are formed in the first two to four years post birth. These attachments set the template for how an individual will build relationships and connections with others throughout their life. Attachment patterns may also inform how people build relationships with animals. These may drive some to have overly close bonds or intense feelings for animals leading to problems for them, for others, and for the animals involved. An example of this may be a person who won't allow an animal to be euthanised even when it is very necessary and is in the animal's best interests. Another example could be those who keep inappropriate numbers of animals, causing welfare issues, including cases which could be considered to be animal hoarding.

Childhood abuse is increasingly recognised as a significant factor in how individuals develop and the few who go on to abuse animals. If people have experienced violence such as beatings as children, then it is very possible this effects how they see the world and they feel that they too need to use such behaviour.

However, others may decide that they will not behave in the same way as adults did with them. They may choose to do something radically different, but they will still be influenced by these early experiences. Monty Roberts might be an example of this. Roberts is a well-known American horse behaviourist. In one of his books, he described how he felt he was treated by his father in ways that were very similar to how horses in the USA were treated and traditionally 'broken' by using harsh and cruel ways in preparation for being ridden. Roberts says he decided that he wasn't going to behave in the same way, rather he was going to use different methods (Roberts 1997). This led him to pioneering new ways to work with horses and becoming internationally well known. He and his wife Pat also went on to foster 47 children, bringing them up very differently to the parenting he experienced. This is an example of how early experiences do not set in stone how we will behave – those experiences can be used to develop and hold a very different frame of reference than the one we were brought up with. However, it is recognised having a trusted adult in our lives as we are growing up will usually be the key to how well we thrive. It doesn't have to be someone obviously significant or with whom we spent a great deal of time – see the example below.

Increasingly, research on the impact of Adverse Childhood Experiences, or ACEs, demonstrates the increased risk of developing problematic behaviours throughout life (Bellis et al. 2014), including violence towards both humans and animals. ACEs, can have a profound neurological impact as brain development in childhood can be impaired by high or chronic stress. This may have consequences on an individual's ability to regulate their emotions, on their cognition or thinking, their memory and learning and upon how they to relate to other people. I suggest that this may, for some people, lead to particularly strong attachments to animals and for others, difficulty in the managing, organising, and planning that is required for good or appropriate animal care. For others, it may cause difficulties with impulse control leading to the acquisition of more animals than can be cared for, managed, or afforded. ACEs can create difficulty in managing emotions that may result for some in violent and cruel behaviour, including to animals.

Box 1.8   Example – ACEs

An example of adverse childhood events (ACEs) was that of a health professional I was teaching who told their story of having a sibling close to them in age. They ended up with very different lives: one a professional, happy and stable; their sibling the opposite. They both experienced ACEs at home as children. There was one simple but hugely impactful difference the settled professional experienced, which her sibling did not. She had a best friend at school whose family accepted her, welcoming her whenever she went around, who gave her somewhere safe to go, and to experience being a part of ordinary family life.

Age: Our age will change our frame of reference. Children see the world in certain ways, not always accurately, which changes as they learn to be more independent of parents or primary carers and move into adolescence. We know that teenagers' brains undergo massive redevelopment in adolescence. Whilst this is happening they are more likely to take risks, be impulsive and less able to assess the harms and benefits of certain actions. During adolescence young people often become self-absorbed and can have difficulty in understanding or recognising the needs and feelings of others, and this may include animals at this point. Adolescents are also likely to imitate others' behaviours. As they move into adulthood, all this usually settles down and they regain and develop abilities to be empathic, manage impulsivity and assess risk.

Older people may have a different view of the world and how they and others fit within it. They can be more aware of their own mortality. For example, interestingly, research shows that older owners of companion animals may have less difficult grief reactions when an animal dies than adolescents (McCutcheon and Fleming 2002).

Aspirations: Human aspirations may be simple. Perhaps, to have a better life for oneself and one's family. Obtaining money may be the main way to making that better life possible for many. Therefore, an individual's aspirations will inform their frame of reference. If animals feature in these aspirations it can affect the ways in which they are treated. Aspirations may be linked to achievements as outlined earlier; people may use their animals in an attempt to make their aspirations bear fruit in the form of achievements. Some of my work has looked at equine welfare cases which involved multiple animals. In some cases those breeding, operating studs, and others, were often 'chasing the one' (Williams et al. 2020) and for many, their aspirations were not realistic. Countless animals could be harmed in the process of their attempt to attain something that was just not achievable.

In wealthier countries, the idea of having an animal or animals can be very appealing. Individuals with disposable incomes can launch into animal ownership with little or no knowledge of the care, time, resources, and possible pitfalls involved. People can see animal ownership or even animal rescuing as a nice idea, but they may lack understanding of the reality. During the Covid-19 pandemic and various lockdowns, many people chose to have companion animals, especially dogs, for the first time. This significantly increased demand for puppies and unscrupulous breeding leading to welfare issues and heartache for new owners. While this may be no more than aspiration and naivety, animals and their welfare inevitably suffer in many of these cases. Aspirations may not have lived up to the hard realities of new pet ownership, especially as lockdowns and restrictions ended and owners returned to the workplace and were able to take holidays again. Several years on from the start of the pandemic, it was recognised that the increase in first-time animal ownership generated a number of different welfare issues. Then a cost-of-living crisis occurred, leading to significant difficulties for some owners and their animals, and the hard reality replaced aspirations.

Hobbies and Interests: In many modern cultures, animals, especially companion animals, are a main hobby or interest for people. This could include dog agility, breeding, showing, or competing, for example. For many people, these types of hobbies can also bring social contact, a sense of pleasure and achievement, all of which is important for human mental health.

Likes and Dislikes: Our likes and dislikes are very personal and can be driven by many other factors in the frame of reference. It is very common for people to be attracted to keeping one type of animal breed and to focus on keeping that breed alone. Many of us will keep the same breeds of companion animals throughout most of our lifetime. Some choose to keep or have a preference for one gender of their chosen species: some horse owners will never want to own a mare and others never a gelding. My research into the hoarding of animals highlighted that it is not uncommon for those who are hoarding to do so with, not only particular species, but also specific breeds. Sometimes, those who hoard keep more than one species but specific breeds of each, for example, Arab horses and Oriental cats. At times, in hoarded situations, some animals are kept in better conditions than others – an example would be when mares were kept in a much better state than stallions or vice versa.

Cultural Influences: For many people, cultural influences colour their world view. These may be traditions that have been handed down over many generations that allow an individual to be a part of a group or family. Individuals can see and then emulate how others, perhaps those who are older or more influential, do things.

Traditions handed down through generations may be deemed important to maintain, even if no longer useful or helpful. For some, there may be religious influences which colour their view of the world. An example may be cow shelters or *gaushalas*. In India's three main religions of Hinduism, Buddhism, and Jainism cows have religious significance, and thus, they are not to be slaughtered. Cow shelters take in old, diseased, or abandoned cows to live out the rest of their lives. The non-slaughter of cattle practices in India means that non-productive or no longer 'useful' animals can be abandoned on the streets by their owners, often being left to scavenge for food. This creates risks and fatalities to both the cattle and humans. The *gaushalas* that take cows in can also have their own animal welfare, human, and environmental consequences.

In the Western world, cultural influences lead to trends and fashions that come and go, and these can apply to companion animals as much as they do to inanimate objects. In the UK, the fashion for 'new' breeds of dogs has been with us for some time. These 'designer' dogs are often crosses of recognised breeds, and some unscrupulous breeding through puppy farms creates much suffering for the animals involved and heartache for those who unwittingly buy them. The Kennel Club warns that the crossing of breeds can exacerbate inherited health problems for each of the breeds. 'Handbag'-sized dogs favoured by celebrities and much publicised by individuals and the media create an aspiration for some – that to achieve the lifestyle of those they admire and follow on social media, they too should acquire a similar animal.

1.4.4   One Other Increasingly Impactful Factor in Our Frame of Reference: Technology

One factor that doesn't appear in the frame of reference is technology. However, technology and social media are something most people now have access to and use regularly. The Internet and social media provides so much information, but we need to know how to assess and critically appraise the sites and pages used and the content and information presented itself.

Box 1.9   Example

For example, a Facebook group that I joined many years ago is dedicated to equine Cushing's disease (PPID). This group greatly helped me understand some of the complex issues around the disease and its management. The moderators were quick to police and call out unproven, unscientific posts and claims by people on the group pages. Through ceaseless monitoring, the administrators of this very large international group are able to check information posted and commented on against the recognised evidence base.

The Internet allows access to peer-reviewed, gold standard open access research papers and to have online conversations with leading experts in a field via social media platforms. It allows us to sign up for massive open online courses (MOOCs) and receive training and education in our own homes from the experts in particular fields and subjects. We can listen to guest lectures and webinars and TED Talks just by signing up or through a quick a Google search, often for free. There are Facebook pages and groups set up to support owners who have animals with specific issues. Never was so much information available for so many people, and animal welfare is well served by all this easily accessible information.

However, the flip side of this is that, as with other areas of life, false information can be easily disseminated quickly and without the person sharing it scrutinising or appraising it. Even worse is that people who wish to profit from others' fears and difficulties can sell unproven and often downright harmful products, techniques, and services. It is easy for well-meaning people to jump on to what looks like a good idea and to support it, and thus, the picture becomes very complex on social media. When an idea or a product is liked, endorsed, or argued for by large numbers of people, it suddenly looks believable. This has been never more evident than in the variance in information in most recent years around human vaccination.

Those purporting to be rescues or sanctuaries can quickly garner support and even funding via social media. In many cases this allows those who are profiting from animal welfare issues, but are unregulated, to attract money and support. This can even support the development of animal hoarding situations.

The Internet enables people to 'investigate' perceived animal welfare situations themselves and quickly publicise them. This can lead to huge harm to innocent individuals or groups who are not committing animal welfare offences or where there are no issues. Such use of technology and social media can adversely affect recognised and legitimate agencies' investigations and interventions in animal welfare cases.

Box 1.10   Helpful Questions to Help Appriase Information

Perhaps we should ask ourselves the following questions:

How does technology impact our view of the world and help us form and change our beliefs?

How do you ensure that you use information from the Internet and from social media wisely?

Reflect about the last piece of information you shared with colleagues, friends, or others via social media. Were you absolutely sure of its provenance?

How do you decide what to share and what not to? How do you scrutinise information?

Lastly, do you think that some people have a lesser ability to scrutinise information in the public domain on social media and other electronic sources and what impact might this have?

1.5   Conclusion

This chapter has explored individual frames of references and what may influence and help create them. The factors described give us our own unique and individual view of the world or the lens through which we see it. Each person has their own backstory and reasons for being as they are or for acting as they do. I have tried to give examples for some of the areas that influence our frame of reference, but you may have others that you can add.

A person's unique frame of reference will be the key to how they think, feel, and behave, and this will include their behaviours with the animals they have or are involved with. To assist someone in making changes, we will need to understand and explore their experiences.

Box 1.11   Exercise

If this chapter has been of use to you, you may want to explore a little more by asking a friend, colleague, or even family member to work with you to explore their frame of reference and how all the factors outlined impact where they find themselves in relation to animals.

If you want, you can use this exercise to also practice your active listening skills that are covered in Chapter 5.

If you do use this exercise, notice what detailed information you gain from the other person, how they may differ from you and perhaps, even though you may know the person well, what new information comes to light that might surprise you.

In the following chapters, the approaches and techniques described for helping people to make changes all rely on an understanding that each person we work with has unique and sometimes profound and unexpected reasons for doing what they do, as well as for why they may or may not decide to make behaviour changes. Being open to understanding the importance of individual experiences, the person's frame of reference, while not necessarily agreeing with them, but hearing and understanding, is going to be crucial.

References

Bellis, M., Hughes, K., Leckenby, N., Perkins, C. and Lowey, H. (2014) National Household Survey of Adverse Childhood Experiences and Their Relationship with Resilience to Health-Harming Behaviours in England. *BMC Medicine.* 12, 72. https://bmcmedicine.biomedcentral.com/articles/10.1186/1741-7015-12-72 (accessed 2.4.2020)

Covey, S. (1989) *The 7 Habits of Highly Effective People. Powerful Lessons in Personal Change.* London: Simon & Schuster UK Ltd.

Dodman, N.H., Brown, D.C. and Serpell, J.A. (2018) Associations between Owner Personality and Psychological Status and the Prevalence of Canine Behavior Problems. *PLOS ONE.* 13, e0192846, https://doi.org/10.1371/journal.pone.0192846.

McCutcheon, K.A. and Fleming, S.J. (2002) Grief Resulting from Euthanasia and Natural Death of Companion Animals. *Omega.* 44, 2, 169–188.

Roberts, M. (August 1997). *The Man Who Listens to Horses.* London: Random House.

Schiff, J. and Schiff, A. (1975). Frames of reference. *Transactional Analysis Journal* 5 (3).

Serpell, J. (2004) Factors Influencing Human Attitudes to Animals and Their Welfare. *Animal Welfare.* 13, 145–151.

Williams, B., Harris, P. and Gordon, C. (2020) What is Equine Hoarding and Can 'Motivational Interviewing' Training be Implemented to Help Enable Behavioural Change in Animal Owners? *Equine Veterinary Education.* 34, 1, 29–36.

2

Behaviour Change – Traditional Methods and Other Ways to Support Behaviour Change in Others

2.1 Introduction

The previous chapter looked at the many experiences and factors that influence people and their view of the world, or their frame of reference. This very personal view will affect individuals' values, attitudes and behaviours, including beliefs and actions where animals are concerned. This chapter explores behaviour change and some of the approaches traditionally used but which don't generally work. Yet, these traditional approaches are what we most often use when attempting to get other people to change their behaviour.

2.2 Traditional Methods Used to Try to Get People to Change Their Behaviour

First, think about the behaviours that you may want those you work with to change for the welfare of their animals. These behaviours may be some of those listed or there may be others, and some may be very specific to your area of work, country, or the culture.

- Feeding appropriately for the animals including not over- or underfeeding
- Water
- Hoof care
- Treating illness and disease
- Responding to animal emergencies
- Seeking veterinary attention

Practical Human Behaviour Change for the Health and Welfare of Animals, First Edition. Bronwen Williams.
© 2024 John Wiley & Sons Ltd. Published 2024 by John Wiley & Sons Ltd.
Companion website: www.wiley.com/go/williams/human

- Maintaining treatment plans including medication
- Vaccinating
- Worming
- Castration
- Breeding
- Harnessing
- Exercise
- Appropriate work /workload including rider weight
- Compassionate handling
- Appropriate care for elderly animals
- Signing over to a charity
- Euthanasia

Box 2.1   Exercise

Now spend a few minutes thinking about how we usually try and enable people to make changes in their behaviour for the well-being or the welfare of animals.
What methods or ways of intervening or taking action have you used or use?
What have you seen or heard your colleagues do?
How does your employer / company / organisation attempt to do this?

When we want people to change behaviours for the benefit of human health or for animal welfare, even with our friends or colleagues we use some well-worn traditional methods. You may recognise some of the methods mentioned below. If you have children, you may have used these at some point to try and get them to make some sort of change. You may even have employed these methods with other family members, including your partner or your parents as they age.

'Traditional' methods we use to try to get people to change

Tell
Advise
Explain
Persuade
Scare / frighten
Educate into submission
Bribe
Emotionally blackmail
Prosecute / use legal action or use it as a threat

Box 2.2   Exercise

Now think about a behaviour that you changed.
It can be a behaviour that you changed recently or one that you changed in the past. It could be one that you changed and then went back to or one that you attempted many times. It could be something such as quitting smoking, eating better, reducing fat or salt in your diet, getting more exercise, reducing the amount of alcohol you consume, having more time away from work, having a better sleep regime or something else.
Now think about what made you change.
Was it other people doing any of those 'traditional' things?
Very possibly not. Change in human behaviour comes about by something that is intrinsic or internal to that person. Simply telling someone they need to change doesn't work.

Traditional methods don't work when we try to get others to change behaviours, just as they don't work when others use them with us. There needs to be another way of supporting people to make changes.

But first, let's look a little more at those traditional methods.

2.2.1   Telling

Often, it is very easy to see what someone else needs to do to make a change that would make life better for them, for others, or their animals. When we are outside a situation or not so personally invested in it, it can appear very clear, if not totally obvious, what needs to be done. However, for the individual, a situation is often more complex and difficult and their frame of reference or worldview (Chapter 1) may be different to ours. They also may not have the skills or belief that they can make a change. Imagine you have a friend who needs to change a behaviour. Perhaps it is quitting smoking or reducing weight. We might say something like...

> 'But if you do this, then you would be so much happier... fitter... healthier... financially better off...'

When we give advice like this, we are often 'stealing all the best lines' (which is covered at 2.3 in this chapter but also see 4.9).

2.2.2   Advising

Just like telling, it is easy to advise. We can do this much of the time. We may have roles where we are employed to give advice; so that is what we do. It is easy to believe we haven't done our job properly if we don't give advice: after all, that is why the client has come to us or why we have been asked to see the owner or visit the animals concerned.

Think about a time when you told someone about an issue you had or something you needed to change. Almost always, the response is for the other person to give advice, to suggest, and often to inform you about what you should do or what they would do or have done in the past. Think about how you felt, especially when you were not actually asking for advice – you were probably not that receptive. But, when other people tell *us* about problems or issues or things they need to change – we give unsolicited advice. Being given unsolicited advice is generally not what we want, and it can be similarly unwanted when we give it to others.

Therefore, just as we are often not seeking advice or guidance, good ideas, or suggestions, other people don't generally want it from us, unless they specifically ask for help, information, or guidance.

At best, giving unwanted advice will stop the individual from sharing information, thoughts, and feelings with us. People can just shut down in conversations. At worst, it will generate difficult feelings, including anger, frustration, irritation or make the person feel disempowered or unable to solve their own problem. It may even have the opposite effect of the well-meant intention and cause the person to move away from wanting or even thinking about making a change. So, we can see that this traditional method of advising, like many of the others, can cause people to be less willing to consider changing, not more. Yet, we still use these traditional techniques when they may be detrimental and have the opposite effect of what we intended.

You may hear someone say to another who is looking to lose weight,

> '*Many people like you have made a change by combining exercise with eating fewer calories and aiming for 2 lbs weight loss a week...*'

Most of us, when we are considering losing weight, already know this!

2.2.3 Explaining

Like telling and advising, we can explain to someone why they *should* make a change. When they don't seem to get it, are not willing to change or do not alter or amend things as fast as we think is required or in the way that we think best, we try explaining to them. We can do this by repeating ourselves and trying to argue in favour of change. When the individual isn't doing what we want or is not receptive to our good advice, we may start to speak more slowly, more clearly, and even more loudly. The same behaviour can be observed when tourists, often

English-speaking ones, who don't know the native language, try to be understood –
they speak more loudly and slowly, as if doing that will make others understand
them. Just as someone doesn't understand when there is a language barrier,
doing this with someone about their behaviour change and our ideas about what
they should do is unlikely to work.

2.2.4   Try to Persuade

When we use persuasion, we are starting to try and use more leverage to move the
person towards change. This, like the previous methods, is probably futile. Yet
we try it.

> Example – *'I know you can do it, just give it a try... You will be happier /
> wealthier / healthier when you do.'*

2.2.5   Educate into Submission

Giving information and trying to educate someone when the time is not right, is
very rarely useful to them. Often, we include lots of information that they
already know, isn't relevant to them, they cannot understand, or is just too
overwhelming.

There *is* a time for giving information when it can be received well, but we need
to skilfully judge when this is. We will look at this 'when' in the coming chapters,
especially in the Stages of Change (Preparation Stage 3.5). There is also a simple
and useful model for giving information when the time is right that can be
found at 9.7.

Perhaps, think about a time when you were given an information leaflet by
your doctor or nurse that you didn't request. How much of it did you read,
if any? Did it just end up in the recycling? There is a time and a place when
information giving can be effective and useful, but carpet-bombing information
doesn't work.

Box 2.3   Quick Exercise
Think how you would respond if, without you requesting it, a doctor or nurse said the following to you while handing over a bunch of paperwork, what would you think and do? 'Let me give you these leaflets about how important diet is and the need to maintain a healthy weight'.

2.2.6 Bribe

Bribery is another traditional method we might use to try to get someone to make a change. Anyone with children in their lives has probably attempted this more than once, often in desperation and when under stress or short of time. We may all recognise this, *'If you don't stop hitting your sister right now, you won't get to choose an ice cream to take home'*.

This method doesn't work well when used with adults, but still, we may give it a go. Many years ago, a good friend of mine, who cared about my health, suggested that if I stopped smoking and didn't smoke for a year, he would give a donation to an equine charity I was involved in. It was a nice offer, and meant kindly, but did I stop smoking then? You can probably guess that the answer was – absolutely not! I would have happily given the donation myself, or a larger one, and continued smoking.

Box 2.4   Exercise

Perhaps, over the next few days, listen out for conversations where someone is being told, advised, informed, or persuaded that something would be better for them.

Listen to the individual's responses and see if you can spot if they start to voice the reasons why change won't work.

Listen to people moving towards or away from change in what they say.

2.2.7 Emotional Blackmail

Like the example of my friend bribing me, using emotional blackmail to get someone to change is often well meaning and driven by concern, care, or love. We may hear someone say, *'But if you cared about me, then you would make this change'*. Or, *'If you want the best for your pet...'*

If it is a human health behaviour we are concerned about, we can use worries about the individual becoming ill or even dying and communicate that concern using emotional blackmail. Although emotional blackmail is unlikely to work on us, we will try it with others. In animal welfare work, emotional blackmail is often used by friends and families who are desperate for a change to be made. It is not unusual for partners or children, often living in the same environment, to try to use emotional blackmail. It rarely works.

In animal welfare, workers may, with the best of intentions, try emotional blackmail in a more covert way: *'You say you care about your animals and if that is the case, you can prove that by making these changes that we need you to make'*. If a change *is* made in situations like this, it will be partial, brief, or inconsistent – to placate others. This is called 'cheap change' (3.4) where someone tries a change without consideration or preparation. In the long term, it can make matters far worse as owners can become secretive and unlikely to ask for information or seek help.

2.2.8 Intervene Practically

Often what needs doing for something to change seems so obvious to us! Not only can we step in verbally but sometimes we do so practically too. We can have a desire to make everything good, to help the person or, in many of our cases, the animals as well as the owner. Miller and Rollnick (2023) describe what they call the 'fixing reflex' where helpers and workers are driven to help and intervene in some way. Most of us have a fixing reflex driven by good intentions. I am often reminded of the story of someone seeing an older person standing by the side of the road looking one way and then the other. A helpful person spots this and motivated by their 'fixing reflex', they take the older person's arm with one hand and with the other, stop the traffic and try to forcefully steer them across. Only to be berated as the person they were helping didn't require their help and is offended! Think about feeling frustrated by a family member or friend when you are trying to support them to do something – often it is easier just to say,

> *'Oh, give it here! Let me do it!'*

Working in animal welfare, health, or care, means we are very likely practical people. Our beliefs about our responsibilities in these roles may well be that to help people and their animals, we must always be able solve problems, make decisions, and make things happen. Our very roles may support and increase our 'fixing reflex' response.

Box 2.5   Exercise

Briefly think about what others expect from you in your work.
   The clients or owners
   Your colleagues
   Your employer or organisation
   And – you
Is there an expectation or are there multiple expectations that drive, reinforce, or increase the fixing reflex for you?

2.2.9 Scare / Frighten

Another traditional method many workers can fall into using, especially when feeling worried or frustrated about the situation, is to attempt to scare or frighten the person into changing.

In animal welfare, this method may be used when we are stuck or out of our depth, or need people to change rapidly, or we are tired. We might say, 'If your animal gets another episode of this, it is likely to die and then how will you feel?' In animal welfare situations, owners may experience this when others around them threatening to involve agencies: *'I could report this to the police or law enforcement and your animals would be taken away'.*

Box 2.6   Saying I Will Change, and then Not Changing

Sometimes, when these traditional methods are used in an effort to get some-one to make a change, we hear them say, 'Yes, yes. OK'. Then, they don't do what is expected of them, or not consistently or for long enough, or they don't come back or take our calls. A person may say yes to what is suggested just to get us off their backs or maybe to be polite. We can then consider the person as dif-ficult or non-compliant or we form some other negative view of them and their behaviour. We lay the blame firmly with them, as we did our best and now they have ignored us. This can lead to feelings of frustration, anger, and even hopelessness in workers.

Box 2.7   Example of Scare Being Unhelpful

At the start of the Covid-19 pandemic, I 'helpfully' sent information to a smoking friend about how much more severe the virus was for those who smoked. And I told them in the message that the World Health Organization had asked me to pass it on to them, which was of course a lie. The fact that this friend had a PhD in their field of expertise still didn't deter me from trying to frighten or scare them into stopping smoking as I *knew* it was the best thing for them. I wanted the best for them, I cared and wanted them to stop smok-ing! Of course, it had absolutely no effect, apart from causing annoyance and making them less likely to come to me for support when they finally do decide to stop smoking.

2.2.10   Prosecute / Use Legal Action or Threaten This as an Outcome

For those working in animal welfare, this may be the last option when everything else has been tried. For some workers, this may indeed be the first option that they use or threaten to use. It is absolutely the first option to use when welfare conditions are such that immediate change and intervention is required. However, even when we have to move to prosecution or legal methods that could lead up to prosecution, such as Improvement Notices in the UK (Animal Welfare Act 2006), these methods may make a difference with only some people, and when they do, it is often only for a short time.

The methods that are outlined and described in this book can still be used in difficult and even hostile situations, including when significant actions and interventions need to be taken, including the use of the law and removal of animals. It isn't that *either* strict enforcement methods *or* different behaviour change approaches should be used. Rather, the two can be used together.

It is not unusual for workers to describe using a 'good cop, bad cop' approach where one worker is softer and more empathic and the other harder and tougher. The approaches that we will consider in this book do not support taking either a 'hard' or 'soft' approach; rather, they allow for something different, an approach that is more helpful to all involved and has much better outcomes, in both the short and the long term.

Prosecution can give agencies and individual workers a sense of purpose and role satisfaction, perhaps of a job well done or completed, and of obtaining 'justice' for the animals involved. Job satisfaction is essential for workers in any role, as is a sense of purpose for individuals and organisations. However, the sad fact is that many animal welfare cases do not reach court in the UK for various reasons. Those that do, including those which result in requirements placed upon the owners including fines and bans, often make little difference to the behaviours of those prosecuted. Many owners who are fined, and even banned from keeping animals, continue regardless with their behaviours.

When our ideas and interventions are at odds with the person who we are trying to help to make change, it causes what Miller and Rollnick (2023) call 'discord'. Discord is caused by the presence of friction in the relationship, a difference of opinion, a lack of understanding of each other's viewpoints. Discord is often subtle, but it can be generated swiftly and become very apparent, especially when a person feels they are not being listened to or that their issues or knowledge are not being acknowledged and appreciated. We will consider discord in more detail in the following chapter (3.8).

2.3 Stealing All the Best Lines

We may list for the person all the good reasons *why* they need to make a change. We tell them what the benefits of change would be, for them, for their animals, for others. We use these in a generally futile attempt to persuade them to make change. We steal all the best lines, leaving the person with few or no good reasons to make change that they can voice.

However, humans are slightly perverse. We have good reasons for doing or not doing things, and for making poor decisions. These background reasons were explored in more detail in Chapter 1 with the frame of reference. Humans also generally want a sense of control over their lives and what they do in it. Therefore, if someone tells a person all the good reasons why they should make a change, it then leaves very little for the individual to talk about other than all the reasons for not changing or what would be problematic about the change or what is good about how things are right now. Stealing all the best lines can even strengthen the person's position of *not* changing. Even if they had been considering making a change, this sort of conversation, where all the best lines are stolen by someone else, can lead the individual to move away from change.

Box 2.8   Example

Humans often love to talk about the need to lose weight, and this may be an example of what can happen when a friend or colleague steals all the best lines.

Friend 1: 'I'm thinking I really need to diet as my clothes are fitting less well!'
Friend 2: 'Have you tried the grapefruit cabbage fasting diet? It really worked for me.'
Friend 1: 'I don't like cabbage.'
Friend 2: 'Well, you could spice it up so you don't notice it was there.'
Friend 1: 'I'm not too keen on grapefruit either.'
Friend 2: 'How about joining a diet club – they worked wonders for my friend.'
Friend 1: 'I don't have the time; I work long hours.'
Friend 2: 'You just need to cut out snacks and refined carbohydrates and sugars.'
Friend 1: 'My life wouldn't be worth living without chocolate. I'm going to buy some bigger clothes! And some bigger bars of chocolate!'

Thus, we can make things even worse and change less likely if we use traditional methods – including stealing all the best lines. So, telling and advising, especially when we steal all the best lines, can make someone less likely to change than they were before our conversation with them.

Think about when you were a child and you complained that you were bored. Adults around you probably gave you lots of really good suggestions about what you might do. If you were like me, you would argue why each of these very good ideas were no use. So much so that none of the options had any appeal at all and you were even more bored. If we had thought up those options ourselves, or been supported to do so, at least one or more would have been enticing.

Box 2.9   Example

Research has shown that over half of us either do not do exercises prescribed to us by physiotherapists or don't do them consistently. I often quote this in training, and when we have physiotherapist participants, they smile and nod. They know this. They are well aware when they work with us, often over a number of sessions, that we won't do what they tell us to do. I really admire physios. They keep on helping their fellow humans. They give important information, that is evidence-based, effective and which often doesn't actually take much time and effort, despite knowing that over half of their clients won't do what they prescribe. The good news is physios working with humans easily pick up the ideas we teach in Motivational Interviewing courses and even manage to increase the success rate with their clients.

2.4   What Has Been Found to Work to Support Behaviour Change: Behaviour Change for Human Health and for Animal Health, Care, and Welfare – Similarities

Motivational interviewing (MI), which is the basis for much of this book, came about through the work of two psychologists, William Miller from the USA and Stephen Rollnick from the UK. MI grew from conversations they had starting in 1982 about their work with those with substance misuse problems, who had been 'sent' for treatment or required to do so by court orders.

Working with those with substance misuse issues has always been difficult. Many of the traditional methods to supporting change outlined in this chapter are often the approaches used by workers, friends, families, and others for those with substance misuse issues. Those with alcohol or drug problems are often told that they need to be 'ready' to change and to be 'motivated'. Then, when the traditional methods don't work and changes haven't been made, they are told to go away and come back when they are ready to change.

Miller and Rollnick realised that for the most difficult behaviours to change, certain approaches with people worked better than others. By having a conversation and trying to understand the person's experience and perspective, change was more likely to come about. It could be said that through these supportive, enquiring conversations, workers were trying to understand the individual's frame of reference or worldview (Chapter 1). These MI interventions supported people to explore their situation and to generate ways to change for themselves. This is the key to change. We know, as outlined earlier, traditional methods for change don't work when they are applied to us and don't work when we use them on others. Helping people to identify themselves what changes are needed and why, and then how to go about them, works so much better.

Interestingly, William Miller came across Monty Roberts and his work. Miller and Roberts have had conversations about how the different ideas and theories they identified are compatible and overlap in many ways: Miller from the world of human psychology and behaviour change and Roberts from his equine behaviour and humane handling area of expertise. Monty Roberts wrote about his meetings and conversations with William Miller in *Horse Sense for People* (1997), and similarly, William Miller wrote a paper about his reflections on the similarities between the two approaches (Miller 2000).

Some of the parallels that Miller identified between Robert's humane handling techniques and MI were that both are about facilitating change; for Roberts change in horses, and for Miller, change in humans. Both approaches encourage working collaboratively (4.10.1) to support the human or animal to find the ways that they can make the change rather than being forced into it. Both methods are non-coercive, based on respect and finding a common 'language' with the other. Both animal handlers or workers with humans need to be flexible, have a relaxed stance, and go 'with their client' when they switch back and forth away from and then towards change. Both types of workers let the animal or the human do the majority of the work. To do this the worker alters their own behaviour moment to moment. Miller and Rollnick (2013) describe this flexible adaptation in the moment as 'dancing' with the client rather than 'wrestling' (see 4.10.1). The traditional approaches to behaviour change outlined above could be seen as 'wrestling'. MI and the other methods to support people to make changes outlined in this book aim for us to 'dance rather than wrestle' with those who need to make changes. Miller and Rollnick's MI approach has been used across many different areas and disciplines as well as countries, cultures, and languages, where human behaviour change needs to be addressed (see 4.5 and 4.10).

Box 2.10   Example – Using Monty Robert's Ideas in an Acute Mental Health Ward

In the mid-1990s, I was a ward manager of a busy mental health admission ward. Those that came to us were often detained under the Mental Health Act, so they were there neither voluntarily nor happily. Sometimes, we needed to make interventions including, as a last resort, the use of physical restraint when the immediate risk of harm to the individual or others was great or when there was absolutely no other way to give medication. For those who have not been involved in acute psychiatry, this can sound horrifying and barbaric, but sometimes, when caring for those who are most acutely unwell, there can be no other option. This type of setting and those events may seem the least likely time and place to use collaborative methods to support someone to facilitate their own change. However, often in those situations, I thought about Monty Roberts' use of the round pen into which a horse was brought to work. Its parameters were very limited within which the animal had to stay with the handler, even though all its instincts were to be out and gone. Similarly, my patients could feel very enclosed and trapped with us, both physically and psychologically. But good nursing, like Roberts' techniques, could still give choice and flexibility wherever possible, even in the smallest of ways. During a physical intervention, if I was the member of the team talking to the patient, I would try to find ways that we could work together to find choices, no matter how small for them. I would talk to them about how 'we' could work together to get us all out of the situation. It didn't always work, but it had better outcomes overall and allowed continued respectful and caring relationships that were a little less traumatising for the individual afterwards. It also helped me, as a nurse, stay connected to the individual and to be as therapeutic as I could be even in situations that I greatly disliked but had responsibility for.

Areas and organisations that use MI include correctional institutions, such as prisons and probation services as well as child safeguarding work. This may be useful to consider when we look at the transfer of behaviour change skills and models to the area of animal health but especially animal welfare. In animal welfare, the focus is on the well-being of the animals involved. It can be difficult to see how these ideas and methods used with humans can be transferred to situations where interventions can include removing animals, euthanasia, the use of legal frameworks, or prosecution.

In the case of probation, there will be a responsibility on the worker to ensure that court orders are carried out by the offender, and when that doesn't happen, they will be required to report back to the court often leading to more severe consequences for the individual. Probation officers and those working in child safeguarding will, as a central part of their jobs, be required to write reports on their clients to be shared with other agencies and with the clients themselves. At first look, there is a massive power imbalance between these workers and those who are required to engage with them. It might be hard to see how these workers could also harness behaviour change methods alongside their rigid responsibilities, enforcement roles and risk assessment and management, while their main focus is always the safety of others such as the general public, children, or other vulnerable people. However, these areas of practice can demonstrate that MI can be used successfully, even when there is a lot at stake and legal frameworks may be in force or at risk of being used. These extreme situations still allow collaborative relationships to be made, in the moment, to help those involved to regain some ability for autonomy and control even when it seems least likely.

If the examples of human health care seem a long way from your work, perhaps think about the skills that good animal workers have. Those who work with animals are tuned into small changes in the animals they are with; for example, being open to tiny clues about discomfort, levels of pain and its location. I suggest those who are used to working with animals and to reading non-verbal signs and tiny clues can be excellent at working with humans and using MI. MI requires attention to tiny details and tuning into the other person, to pick up fine shifts in one direction and then another. Just like Monty Roberts, who goes with these small changes and when there is a move towards change reinforces it, so it can be when we work with humans to make changes.

2.5   The Increasing Interest in Behaviour Change for the Good of Society

There is increasing interest in how humans change behaviours. Many people come to our MI training courses with the expectation that they will come away with skills that will enable them to *make* other people to change behaviour. This is understandable and it occurs in courses both for those working in human health and for those working in animal health, care, and welfare. We all would like the silver bullet, the quick fix, a sure-fire way of getting others to do what we need them to do, for their best interests, the best interests of their animals, other people and even us. We come to courses, and to books like this one, looking for answers. This is because, at some level, we recognise that the traditional methods just aren't working; so we look for a new approach. However, we assume there must be another 'secret' traditional method out there, but we just don't know about it.

The reality is we can't make other people change, just as no one can make you or I change. This is why the traditional methods don't really work. People at first often look quite deflated, disappointed, and perplexed when we say this in our courses.

Box 2.11   Society-wide Behaviour Change

Governments and health and social care departments at local, national, and international levels have become very interested in recent years in the psychology of behaviour change. It is recognised that for many of us our lifestyle, especially a Western one, has become sedentary with high calorie, fat, sugar, and salt intake. Add in alcohol and tobacco use and it gets worse.

Consequently, although we are living longer than our forefathers and even the generation before us, we are developing significant health issues, especially those linked to obesity, diabetes, cancers, chronic lung disease, stroke, and coronary heart disease. Now, in many populations, there is increasing comorbidity where individuals suffer several of these diseases at the same time, thus impacting their physical and mental health, social life, and productivity. It is recognised that chronic disease and deaths are increasing rapidly, especially in low- and middle-income countries. These diseases are expensive to treat and people may live for many years needing increasing levels of care. All of this is costly, and so, perhaps very understandably, governments and national and international organisations recognise this economic impact and have looked at ways to change people's behaviours to reduce the impact of poor lifestyles and the consequent diseases, care, and costs associated with them. A number of different types of approaches have been successful, such as legislation in the UK around the advertising and display of tobacco and cigarettes and a ban on smoking in public places. Other approaches have been national information programmes, some of which are very successful, and some less so.

Poverty and chronic diseases are recognised as a significant issue by the World Health Organisation, and some of the humans we work with in animal health and welfare may be experiencing these. Thus, owners may be unable to access the appropriate human resources even for themselves, or have a lack information and knowledge about how to do so. If that is the case, how difficult then will it be for them to then consider making changes around how they look after their animals? For many readers working in animal welfare, this will already be something you recognise, and, using the 'One Health Approach' many animal welfare organisations are working to improve the health of the humans as well as their animals, recognising that these are intrinsically linked.

One often mentioned idea to support behaviour change in human health is 'nudge' theory. 'Nudging' uses knowledge about human thinking to support behaviour change, by giving people choices that then help them make 'better' ones. The originators of nudge theory, Thaler and Sunstien (2008), describe this by giving examples such as putting fruit on eye level in shops rather than banning junk food, thus supporting better choices through coaxing. A memorable example of the use of nudge theory in action is the men's urinals in Amsterdam's Schiphol Airport where an image of a housefly was incorporated in the bowl to encourage a better 'aim' by those using them.

Nudge theory may be useful to consider for animal welfare and animal health organisations. It, and similar theories, will undoubtedly have a place in these areas, especially when large groups or populations are being encouraged to change. However, what we are looking at with behaviour change, especially the use of MI, in this book is working with individuals or small numbers of people to help them change specific behaviours in ways that are unique to them.

So while human health behaviour can be affected for many in the population with laws and policies, other interventions such as improving access to resources and giving information will also improve things. But there will always be a residual but not insignificant number of people, who, despite all these societal changes and pressures, will continue to make poor choices for themselves leading to chronic diseases.

So it is the same in animal health and welfare work. Large numbers of animal-owning populations can be supported and encouraged to change behaviours through legislation, education, community and societal programmes. There are some though who will not be able to do this, with whom a more individual approach is needed, which many of us do anyway in our day-to-day roles.

Interestingly, the issues that beset a Western lifestyle, that of obesity and chronic diseases, are being replicated in some animal ownership, especially for companion animals. It is increasingly common for dogs and cats and other companion animals to be overweight or obese, to be more sedentary, and so to develop chronic and disabling health conditions including joint disorders, respiratory and heart problems. In the equine world, the issue of overfeeding and underwork is increasingly a welfare issue in the UK leading to an increase in chronic problems including Equine Metabolic Syndrome and also acute and chronic foot disorders.

There needs to be another way, and that is what this book is about. The ideas, models, techniques, and approaches described here are not methods to trick or to make people change their behaviours. It isn't about manipulating people to do what you, or others, believe is best. This is going to be a key idea to grasp, but it is not an easy one.

2.6 Conclusion

This chapter started with the traditional methods that we tend to use to try and get people to change, to be where *we* think they need to be, when we believe we can see what's best and what is needed. The previous chapter (Chapter 1) looked at the

Box 2.12 Exercise

Exercise – Think about the issues below from human health and consider how much matches your animal health and welfare experiences.

Human	Animal
Poor / inappropriate diet	
Over or under calories	
Poor nutritional value	
Lack of exercise	
Overweight / obesity	
Not accessing health checks and screens	
Poor / no management of existing disorders (e.g. diabetes)	
Inconsistent / poor concordance/ compliance with medication	
Not taking up treatment offered / options	
Not doing required physiotherapy exercises	
Not taking up or completing courses of vaccination	

different ways we all see the world, ourselves, and our animals: our frame of reference. We will need to work with people collaboratively, understand them, seeing the world through their frame of reference, not ours, to support changes to be made in ways that are suitable for them. Finally, this chapter has given a brief outline of how important behaviour change for humans is with the impact of modern life on humans. Increasing health and social care costs are leading to a growing interest in behaviour change by many governments and organisations.

In the next chapter, we will look at a well-known theory of how people make behaviour changes, called the 'Transtheoretical Model' or the 'Stages of Change Model'. This can be very useful in aiding understanding about what approaches we might take with people and when to use them. It allows us to offer more useful interventions, and at times that are more likely to support people to make change.

References

Animal Welfare Act. (2006). https://www.legislation.gov.uk/ukpga/2006/45/contents (last accessed 9 September 2023).

Miller, R. (2000) Motivational Interviewing: IV. Some Parallels with Horse Whispering. *Behavioural and Cognitive Psychotherapy.* 28, 285–292.

Miller, W.R. and Rollnick, S. (2023). *Motivational Interviewing: Helping People Change and Grow*, 4th ed. New York: Guilford Press.

Miller, W.R. and Rollnick, S. (2013). *Motivational Interviewing: Helping People Change*, 3rd ed. New York: Guilford Press.

Roberts, M. (August 1997) *The Man Who Listens to Horses*. London: Random House.

Thaler, R.H. and Sunstein, C.R. (2008). *Nudge: Improving Decisions about Health, Wealth, and Happiness*. New Haven: Yale University Press.

3

The Stages of Change Model

3.1 Introduction

The previous chapters have explored how various experiences frame our view of the world and can influence how we act and then how the traditional approaches used to encourage or persuade people to change generally don't work, especially in the medium to long term. Therefore, we need to find other ways to help people make changes. This chapter will outline a widely recognised model about how people make changes which can be useful to underpin our approaches as workers. This model will be used through this book to guide which techniques, or structures, we might be able to employ in interactions with people when they are in different stages of change.

3.2 The Stages of Change Model (or Transtheoretical Model)

The Stages of Change Model, also known as the 'Transtheoretical Model' for human behaviour change, was first developed in the 1980s by psychologists, all now professors, James Prochaska and Carlo DiClemente, along with their colleague John Norcross. Their original research looked at how people made changes and what methods they used to do so. Prochaska, DiClemente and Norcross realised that most people made all sorts of changes, both big and small, throughout their lifetimes. The majority of these changes occurred without specialist interventions or help from people such as psychologists, nurses, councillors, doctors, experts, or other professionals. Most people make changes themselves or are 'self-changers', as Prochaska et al. (1994) described them.

Practical Human Behaviour Change for the Health and Welfare of Animals,
First Edition. Bronwen Williams.
© 2024 John Wiley & Sons Ltd. Published 2024 by John Wiley & Sons Ltd.
Companion website: www.wiley.com/go/williams/human

Box 3.1	Exercise

Take a few minutes to think about changes you have made over time, perhaps over your lifetime.
Maybe write down a few of them.
Now, think about each change that you made. Make a note about whether you did this change yourself (self-change) or whether you had specialist help or other support.
You may identify that all the changes were self-change with no help from a specialist or that perhaps some were self-change and some were with interventions from others.

Change you have made	Self-change?	Help from others?

Most human behaviour change is self-change, for example, most people who stop smoking do so without interventions from others. This doesn't mean that help from those with specific expertise isn't required; rather, it isn't needed all of the time and not for everybody, or for every change. With this knowledge, when we come in contact with people who need to alter their behaviour for the sake of animal health or welfare, we can be hopeful for change. It may be that the person will only need us in certain ways at particular times to support them. Everyone is unique and each behaviour change is different. Sometimes, even making the same behaviour change is different at different times. For example, someone may stop smoking a number of times, using alternative methods for each attempt.

However, when Prochaska et al. (1994) looked at how people had made changes, they were surprised to find that there were similar steps and methods used by many people at certain points in behaviour alteration. This led to the development of the Stages of Change Model, or the 'Transtheoretical Model' as it is also called. Prochaska, DiClemente, and others have continued to research and develop the model, increasing understanding about how people make changes and what they need to be able to do so.

Some critics of the Stages of Change Model point out that it can be wrongly used as an indication of whether or not someone is actually ready to make a change at a particular point in time. Rather, the model needs to be understood and used more subtly, and not as a blunt indicator of readiness to change. It has also been used by some organisations and agencies to demonstrate outcomes, and again, it is suggested that this can be unhelpful and miss the true meaning of the model.

As we shall consider in the following chapters, thoughts and behaviours around change are not simplistic and linear for any individual. Rarely does anyone move from one stage of change to another then to finally making the change and sticking to it. If only it were that simple. In this book, the stages of change are used as a useful guiding framework. It can be used to help us understand how to approach conversations as they ebb away from, and flow towards change.

The Stages of Change Model can be useful for those working in animal health, care, and welfare as it can help us identify which methods would fit best with where the individual is within the stages of change at that moment. Now we will look in more detail at these different stages of change and how they can help when we support someone to change their behaviour for the health or welfare of their animals and sometimes for their own welfare and that of other humans.

The Stages of Change Model

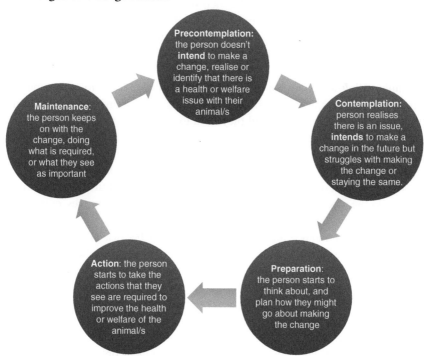

Source: Adapted from Prochaska et al. (1994)

These stages were originally based on addictions, but this model works for many changes humans might make, especially major ones. It suggests that we pass through a number of stages when making a change. One behaviour I often choose to illustrate this is smoking, as it is a really clear behaviour for most of those who smoke, but there are lots of other examples of changes where the Stages of Change Model can be traced.

3.3 Precontemplation Stage

In the precontemplation stage, people have no intention of changing, at least in the foreseeable future. They may even be unaware that there is an issue. Someone who smokes, for example, may not see that there is any issue with their smoking. They might say something like, 'My grandmother smoked all her life, and she died when she was 97 years old... When she fell under a lorry... Smoking never did her any harm!'

The main issue for the individual in this stage tends to be other people's perceptions that there *is* a problem, when they themselves do not see any. For someone smoking, for example, it may be their doctor, their spouse, or other family members who identify the problem or the need for a change. In animal health, for an individual in the precontemplation stage, it may be a veterinary professional, a welfare worker, or a family member who sees there is a problem, but not the owner.

Simply telling someone that they need to make a change, to do something differently, won't work in the precontemplation stage. The individual doesn't think there is a problem, so why should they need to do anything? This links with the traditional methods often used to try to get someone to change outlined in the previous chapter (Chapter 2). Traditional methods of telling, advising, or educating, for example, are of little or no use with someone who doesn't see that there are any issues that need attention right now, or even ever. In human health, those who are in the precontemplation stage may present to doctors, nurses, or councillors, but often, this is because of pressure from others.

Similarly, in animal health, owners may come to us because of concerns raised by someone or because others have told them to contact us. For those working in veterinary and similar settings, owners may present their animals but with little or no thought that they, as the owner, will have to make changes. They may look to workers to prescribe or intervene as the way forward, but not expect they will need to do anything differently. Animal owners in the precontemplation stage may not intend to make a change imminently but may still present their animals just to stop other people nagging them. Despite contacting us or presenting animals to practices they may see no reason why our input might be required.

In animal welfare work, an owner may not see a problem and perhaps just wants welfare workers to go away and stop hassling them, or they may not have any intention to change the behaviour at present.

Owners in the precontemplation stage will probably reject any help, support, direction, advice, or criticism. Why would they need to make a change when they don't intend to change right now or see no reason or don't need to? If you didn't think you needed to make a change in *your* life, or didn't intend to make a change right now, why would you go to all that effort and time to undertake a change merely because others told you to do so?

Some owners may have historically kept animals in a particular way. They, and perhaps their family and community, may have always done it this way. It might be useful to try and see the situation from the individual's point of view or frame of reference (Chapter 1) when they are in the precontemplation stage. If the owner doesn't see that there is a problem, we can ask them why others might believe change is required. We can also ask the owner why they think things *don't* need to be different.

Some people may feel despondent and hopeless about change. What would be the point in considering a change if it seems impossible to even start? The situation might feel so huge that they are not in a position to contemplate or think about change. They might not know how to make the change, or in complex situations, even where to begin. Change could mean so much effort on their behalf that it feels impossible, or that they don't have the ability, or the time or the resources to undertake or even consider it.

For those of us working in animal welfare work, when we meet those in the precontemplation stage, they may be, quite understandably, unhappy to see us. They don't recognise that there is a problem, so why are we there? Perhaps they see us as intrusive, wasting their time and invading their privacy.

Box 3.2   Brief Exercise

Think about how you would react right now if someone came to you to tell you that there was something wrong with your care of an animal and you needed to make changes, when you believe everything is absolutely fine.
How would this be if they arrived at your home or place of work to tell you this? How would you react?
How would your frame of reference (Chapter 1) support or influence your response?

This links back to the *frame of reference* (Chapter 1) and people's beliefs and views of the world. Whilst working in equine welfare, in most of the cases to which I was sent, people were unhappy that someone had reported them. Even at some of the yearly home checks I have done in the past, for animals out on loan from a charity, the guardian can be sometimes unwilling to fully engage. This may well be due to their beliefs and values; perhaps thinking that they have sufficient experience and don't need someone, especially me, coming to check on them. Perhaps, they believed that, as they have been good enough to take on an animal with all the responsibility and expense required, it is a bit of an affront to be inspected. There may be very many other reasons that are not simple, and are unique to that person and their frame of reference.

Box 3.3   Exercise

Can you think of anything at all that you do or don't do currently that you have no inclination to change imminently? Are there other people in your life who may view the situation differently?
Or can you identify someone you know who has no intention of making a behaviour change when others think that they should?

3.4   Contemplation Stage

In the contemplation stage, there is a realisation, understanding, or knowledge that a change is probably required. There may be an intention to change, *but* not right now. This could be because the person is not ready, isn't able, it isn't the right time, it will be too difficult, too expensive, or for other reasons particular to them. Therefore, in the contemplation stage, someone might know that a change needs to be made, but they are not able or perhaps unwilling to do it right now.

Many of us will have said to ourselves that our diet needs to change in some way. The following conversation in our heads may be familiar.

> *I need to lose weight / eat healthier / consume less sugary snacks / consume less alcohol.*
> But we may also think...
> *Christmas / my holiday / anniversary is just around the corner and I want to enjoy that.*

That '*but*' is important. It is pivotal, around which change might happen, or things may stay the same. The *but* is like the middle of a seesaw. In the contemplation stage the individual is moving towards one end of the seesaw, towards thinking about the change and then switching back towards the other end, to keeping the situation as it is, or maintaining the status quo.

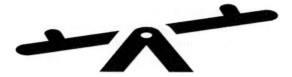

This moving back and forth, between knowing a change is probably needed but not being ready to do it right now, is called 'ambivalence'. We will come back to ambivalence as it is central to behaviour change, especially when using MI approaches (4.9 and 8.1). When we first hear the word ambivalence, it can often be interpreted as someone not being bothered or not caring. In fact it is very different. The person does care, feels two ways about an issue, rather than nothing about it. Ambivalence can be quite an intense feeling and hard to completely dismiss when we have it.

So... someone who smokes might say to themselves (as I did when I smoked),

'I really should stop smoking... soon... but... not today.'

In the contemplation stage, people begin to recognise that there is an issue and to think about the possibility of change. Many of us know, for much of our lives, that we should be changing a behaviour in some way, that it will benefit us, but we are not quite ready to get on with it right now.

People need to have time in the contemplation stage. They require the opportunity to weigh up and move (or not) towards change. Prochaska et al.'s (1994) work with people who smoked found the average time spent in contemplation was around two years before a change was then made. This illustrates that for many changes, especially big behaviour changes, people need time to mull them over.

This two-year contemplation timeframe can be disheartening for workers in both the human health and animal health worlds. Change often doesn't happen rapidly, and people generally need time to experience the discomfort of contemplation and the ambivalence that comes with this stage of change. However, it can help us understand that sometimes it takes time to work with people before they make the change. Some changes can happen faster though. Or we may start working with someone and not realise that they have already been thinking about, contemplating, making a change for some time. Then, with just a little bit of the right help and support, they can quickly move into action and make a successful change.

This can give hope when we are working with owners. It can remind us that it is worth spending time with people who are ambivalent about making change, as they move back and forth with those pivotal, seesaw-type thinking, feelings, and behaviours.

When we talk to someone who is in the contemplation stage of change, whether a client, owner, friend, or family member, it is common to feel frustrated or even useless. It may feel hopeless working with someone when they are ambivalent. In fact, contemplation can be the most fruitful stage for us to help someone move towards change. We just have to provide suitable support for them and for this stage of change. This is what much of the skill in helping people to make successful change is about.

'Shall I change?' / 'Why would I change?'

Sometimes, however, people do change quickly. We know that people will often be more prepared to engage and to perhaps make changes when there is some sort of crisis for them or those around them. This can generate the momentum needed to start to make a change. Change is hard and takes energy, so a crisis can provide the required fuel to drive change.

The other side of this is something that has been called 'cheap change' (see also 2.2.7 and 4.9). We may all recognise cheap change. We wake up and decide that today is the day to start a diet, but we do so without much preparation or thought (or without time in the contemplation or preparation stages of change). Then, a colleague with a birthday brings our favourite cakes to work. Or waking up the day after a celebration we swear we won't drink alcohol again, but then along comes that tempting offer of a drink that we can't refuse. This is why many of us who make New Year resolutions are not successful with them. Without sufficient contemplation with its seesawing of ambivalence followed by sufficient preparation, changes rarely stick.

Making a change is not easy. From the outside, to those around the person, it often looks like it should or could be easily done. Similarly, it is really straightforward to see what needs to be done and how problems can be solved – when they are other people's, not our own. Making a change requires energy, but staying the same, not changing can require less or no effort. Therefore, it is often easier to stay as we are and leave change for another day, another year or decade.

Box 3.4   Example

An example of this might be those who are using drugs such as opiates and find themselves living on the streets, homeless. Passers-by could look at them and see that it is obvious that, by making make some changes they could have a much better life. It seems simple from where we stand outside the experience. It can appear inexplicable why people may continue to behave and live like this despite being offered help, or resources being available to them.

Now, let's think about their situation again, from a different angle. Making a change such as giving up illicit drugs, on which you may well be physically and psychologically dependant, requires a massive change or series of changes.

These changes are hard emotionally and physically; the person may have withdrawal effects, lose their street friends and companions, or be flooded emotionally by memories and feelings that the drugs keep at bay. They probably will have to move areas and start again from scratch. For many who are street homeless, they are very unlikely be able to take their companion animal with them, if they have one, to an accommodation they are offered or to a detoxification and rehabilitation facility. Right now, in the immediate short term, it is easier to find another fix of drugs and live as they are, to keep the status quo. This takes far less energy than starting to make changes. The individual may feel that they have too much to lose by making a change, while other people who are not in their situation would think that they have everything to gain.

Box 3.5   Traditional Methods of Trying to Get Someone to Change Are Like a Salesperson Cold Calling

We are all familiar with someone coming to our door, or calling us, unsolicited. They want us to buy something from them. Cold calling rarely works. The salesperson will need to contact many, many people before they get a sale. When it does work, I think that the person probably already had at the back of their mind that they needed the very item or service being offered. So the salesperson strikes lucky. Or maybe we buy the least expensive thing just to get them off our backs. Or we may even ask them to call back or to send the details and then switch our phones off, block the number, or give an incorrect email address.

This is very similar to how we give unsolicited advice or other interventions to people who may need to make a change and it explains the less-than-good responses we receive when giving that advice.

For some people, their experiences and frame of reference (Chapter 1) may mean that they view themselves as unable to change, or they may feel hopeless. To make a change, we have to have a sense that we can do it with what is called 'self-efficacy'.

Self-efficacy is our belief that change is possible for us. We also have to have a sense of self-worth or self-esteem to feel that it is worth the investment to make that change, spend all that time, energy and effort in something that is for us. If you don't have at least some self-efficacy, self-esteem, and confidence in your abilities, change will seem impossible (for more about self-efficacy, see 11.15 and 12.6, for self-esteem 11.14).

Some people can be stuck in contemplation for years – what Prochaska et al. (1994) described as chronic contemplation where they procrastinate, knowing that they need to make a change but are unable to do it. Several people I know – including myself – were chronic contemplators when smoking. We never were in precontemplation, rather we spent the whole of our smoking careers in contemplation, which didn't really make it very enjoyable. People can feel very powerless when in chronic contemplation.

So, we need to be aware that some people can become stuck in the contemplation stage (chronic contemplation). On the other hand, there is evidence that if people move too quickly through the contemplation stage (with cheap change), they are less likely to succeed with their desired health behaviour change in the long run. This is important to remember when working with animal owners and others. We can become caught up in the excitement of an owner's swift move to contemplation and then we try to push them on into the action phase. People need to be supported in the contemplation stage to allow them to make a well-considered change with sufficient preparation before they move into action. Supporting people in contemplation can also help them to identify that they have been thinking about change for some time and now just need a bit of help to move towards the change. Some people may be stuck in chronic contemplation and we need to be prepared to help them consider starting to move towards change.

Box 3.6   Exercise – Ambivalence

Can you think of a behaviour with which you are currently in the contemplation stage or remember a time when you were contemplating before you made a change? Can you recognise the two sides of your thinking with a 'but' in the middle?

Change I could make ....but...

If you have identified something here, you are seeing ambivalence!
Now – can you think of a time when you rushed into a change without thought or preparation or just to please someone else and it didn't last?
This could be cheap change.
And now, can you identify a behaviour where you have been stuck in chronic contemplation *or think of someone you know who may have been stuck in it?*

Box 3.7   Exercise – Knowing There is a Problem But Being Defensive

Think for a moment about the animals you have in your life. If you are honest, is there something that needs doing that you haven't quite got around to doing? Maybe you have put it off until tomorrow or next week as you are busy? Consider a hypothetical scenario where someone in authority or with particular knowledge about animals is coming to your home or where you keep your animals. What would you do in anticipation of this visit?

For me, it is always that my feed and equipment sheds are never quite as tidy as I think they should be. So, if someone turned up to see my animals unexpectedly, I would be acutely aware of the things I haven't quite done and have let slip. This would probably make me quite defensive and, knowing me, quite vocal with the unexpected visitor! Perhaps this starts to give an idea of how contemplation can work in animal health or welfare issues, especially when our roles require visits to owners. They may be aware in the back of their mind that there are things that need attention, but not immediately. Or they may be aware of issues but could become quite defensive. How then can we help people feel less defensive and start to talk about what they know might be the issues?

If we see owners away from their own environment, they may be in the contemplation stage and yet defensive, knowing that they haven't done as much as they perhaps might have done. For example, an owner may bring a dog to an appointment, knowing that they haven't managed to exercise it as much as they should have during the past few weeks.

As someone makes a shift from contemplation towards preparation, their focus changes from the problem to the solution and from the past to the future (Prochaska et al. 1994). Our listening skills (see Chapter 5) will help us here to pick up fine clues in the person's use of language, we may hear subtle shifts. For example, an owner may start to move from talking about the difficulties of managing an animal's health condition and how it's not worked before to wondering about how they could fund possible treatment. It may not sound like much, but if there is a shift in their language, then there is movement in their thinking about change. We will explore how to develop and use listening skills, essential for helping people to think about and make changes, in Chapter 5. Occasionally, someone in contemplation may ask for advice, guidance, or information. If we offer this, it should be done carefully, if at all at this stage. The judgement will be yours, and it needs to be a carefully considered decision. It can be far more useful and powerful to ask the owner what they think, what they have thought about or tried already, or seen others try or accomplish, before we start giving information. This allows the individual to, if possible, find the answers themselves. If they are able to do this, guided by us, it will make change much more likely, more consistent and long lasting. Chapters 7 and 8 will cover in detail how to work with people in contemplation.

3.5   Preparation Stage

In the preparation stage, an individual begins to really think about the change, to see it as a possibility. They may ask others how to do it or enquire about how someone made a similar change, or they might start gathering information through activities such as reading or watching videos. Here is the opportunity to offer information that might help the person preparing to make a change. This still should be done with care, caution, and judgement. A useful, simple model to support helpful information giving can be found at 9.7 and 9.8.

Someone in the preparation stage may start experimenting (9.2). For example, someone who smokes may experiment by changing their brand of cigarette or by reducing the number of cigarettes smoked each day or have their first cigarette later in the day. I've known people who buy a brand that they absolutely hate when they want to stop smoking. They may set a date to start the change or make plans of how they can go about it. For example, a dog owner might buy some different food to see if their pet likes it, ask a friend if they can walk with them with their dog on a regular basis, or contact a dog walker to see how much they charge. We can see that this looks very different from contemplation.

The individual may devise plans or methods that we don't think will work, won't be successful for change. Here, patience by the worker is needed. If feasible, we need to support the individual to explore all possible methods of change appropriate for them and then consider how to manage any difficulties. More can be found in Chapter 10 about how to do this. Sometimes, we need to let people experiment and discover for themselves that their original methods won't work and other approaches are needed. Our role is, as much as possible, to support and help them develop their confidence and self-efficacy (11.15, 12.6) and to maintain a belief that they can make a change if a first attempt does not turn out as expected.

Prochaska et al. (1994) stated that the preparation stage is essential to successful behaviour change, and it needs to be seen as distinct from the contemplation stage. In contemplation, changing and not changing are thought about. In preparation, decisions are taken to undertake change. The foundations are laid on which to then build change. However, preparation is often ignored or underestimated by other people around the individual, which can cause problems in the next stage – action. Prochaska et al. (1994) cautioned that when the preparation stage is brief and not thought through (or involves cheap change as discussed earlier), the chances of long-term success is reduced.

In the preparation stage, specific steps are identified and firmed up to be put to use in the next stage – action. For someone who smokes, the preparation stage might, for example, include reading about nicotine replacement, making appointments with the GP or smoking cessation nurse, buying patches, setting a date, or cutting down. They may read up on how others have stopped smoking, seek out inspirational videos, or talk to friends or colleagues who have stopped and ask them how they did it.

All may not be simple and straightforward though, because in the preparation stage it is easy to slide back into contemplation or even precontemplation stages. We as workers (or family, friends, or colleagues) can become overly excited when someone is in the preparation stage and believe that we, and they, have cracked it, and change is an imminent certainty! The person needs to be allowed to hesitate, to be cautious, to wonder if now is the time, if there might be a better way or if they shouldn't just leave the change for now.

Goal setting doesn't really work until the preparation stage. Helping people set goals and action plans is how we can be useful here, as well as in helping them to think about what could go wrong, any potential pitfalls, and how they might manage those. Breaking goals down into smaller goals or steps can be really helpful and will support people to increase their self-efficacy (11.15) and allow the change to appear more manageable and achievable. They may need support with skills that they need to succeed. For example, giving medication or treatment to someone for their animals is unlikely to work if the person doesn't have the skills or the knowledge of how to use and administer it. More information about supporting goals development and action planning can be found in Chapter 10.

In your role, you may use training, education, or the giving of information in other ways to owners and others to enable them see that behaviour change is needed. Preparation is the most useful stage of change in which to give information (9.7–9.9). Trying to inform, educate or give information in the precontemplation or contemplation stages is unlikely to work.

Self-efficacy is again important here. Previous changes, and the methods used then, can be identified and used to support the belief that another change is possible (self-efficacy – see 11.15, 12.6). And then, it becomes more worth the effort and the investment to make the change.

Box 3.8 Brief Exercise

Think about a behaviour change you have made recently or in the past, even if you only made the change for a while. What preparation did you do for the change? What helped? And what didn't? What in your preparation had the most impact? If you were to make the change again, what would you do differently in the preparation stage? And if you were to make a different change, what could you learn from this one?

How could you use questions like this to help someone else preparing to make a change?

3.6 Action Stage

In the action stage, people begin to change their behaviour in line with their goals. It may not always go to plan, but they start doing it. Here, in action, people need support to keep going and to move towards maintenance. Action is when you have smoked your last cigarette and either don't buy anymore or, as I did, throw the rest of your cigarettes into the fire. And maybe, you tell your friends, 'Don't offer me a cigarette – as I don't smoke anymore!' There is change in thinking and behaviour – *I have stopped smoking, I am not smoking.*

The action stage is when people actually get on and start the behaviour change. If thinking and planning in the preparation stage has been undertaken sufficiently, individuals will have strategies in place to use in the action phase. One of the big risks in the action stage is that those around an individual believe that their input and support is no longer needed as all is now well because the behaviour has been changed. The reality is that this is the stage in which people really need support to enable continued change and to deal with setbacks and problems as these occur.

How we support people in the action stage of change will be different to the other stages. Adaption of our working style and techniques will be needed to match the stage of change and also the individual. I often see both human health and animal health, care and welfare colleagues drop the support and help given once some change has started. Appointments are reduced or visits stopped. This can be a mistake, as this is often when people really need the help to keep going.

Prochaska et al. (1994) state that it is the action stage that is most visible to others. At this point those making changes get the most recognition from other people, but it is often short-lived. In the action stage, professionals and others may see the person has made the change and think that their work is now done – the person is on the right track and can be left to get on with the successful behaviour change. However, an action stage takes a lot of time, energy, and resources from the individual, and they need input and support in different ways throughout this stage.

Box 3.9   Exercise

Think back to a behaviour change you have made recently or in the past.
How was the action stage for you?
How much energy did it take?
Did other people notice?
If they did, how did they support you?
What helped and what didn't? And if you can, think of two or three behaviour changes you have made (even if they didn't stick or continue) – what worked for you and what didn't, especially in the action stage?

3.7   Maintenance Stage

In the maintenance stage, there is a need to consolidate the change and to work on continuing the new behaviour, but often help from others stops at, or before, this point. Again, they need continued support in this stage. However, input from us doesn't need to be a great deal. What is more important is that support is available and accessible when needed. Think about those of us who used to smoke; people are often very supportive in the first days and maybe weeks, but they soon forget to say well done as often, or at all. However, as time passes, there are still times when we miss those cigarettes, but now we can feel alone and without help. For changes to improve animal health or welfare, support will be needed for owners to make behaviour changes that stick and continue. For more information on the maintenance stage and how to help, see Chapter 12.

For some people maintenance is ongoing for the rest of their lives. For instance, with human health behaviours such as consuming alcohol and other substances, some people will battle with maintaining the change each and every day. They will be building strategies and needing support from others. This can be the same for some animal health and especially animal welfare issues. Some people may continually or intermittently struggle with maintaining changes. An example here would be someone who has urges to take in more animals than they can manage. Perhaps they have a need to rescue and to help animals they see in need. Someone with such feelings and thoughts may have to continue to manage these for months or years or even the rest of their life.

Other people, however, can move to a new reality where the change is embedded and now normal for them. In a later work, Prochaska and DiClemente (1992) added another stage in their model; a final one to which they gave the slightly unfortunate title of termination. Termination stage is where an individual has successfully made the change, so much so that the issue is no longer a part of their life. People become so familiar with the change that the old behaviour is no longer even thought about. They now have difficulty imagining the behaviour ever being a part of their life again in the future. Smoking illustrates this well. Some will find it hard to even recognise that they were the person who smoked and cannot now really believe that they once did so. They may even have an intense dislike of the smell of cigarette smoke. Someone experiencing this may well be in the termination stage of change. For others, not smoking will always be a continual battle that rarely goes away. They may inhale deeply when near someone smoking and look longingly at cigarette packets and associated paraphernalia such as lighters. People experiencing this may continue in the maintenance stage, a very different experience than those who are in the termination stage. A return to smoking could easily happen if they didn't monitor themselves and work to stay a non-smoker.

In animal health and welfare work, this is useful to consider. Many owners can make changes successfully with some initial support and then never need input again. Others, especially some welfare cases, may need some continued support and contact from agencies and workers. This can ensure they are supported in the maintenance stage and do not a slip back, or if they do, it is picked up early and they can be helped to get back on track. For those who work with owners who have behaviours such as hoarding animals, this will be essential.

A key message for workers is that, despite the fact that people making changes need acknowledgement and support in all of the stages, they often don't get it. When working with people who make successful changes, we need to consider who might offer them support and how that might be done for the maintenance of change.

3.8 Discord

Discord was mentioned in the previous chapter (2.2.10). Often, discord occurs when the worker and the owner are not on the same page or in the same place when discussing the behaviour or change needed. Discord happens when individuals are not matched or in the same place in their interactions. There can be a friction, or what I describe as a scratchiness, between them. One way of creating discord is for there to be a mismatch between where the owner is in the stages of change at a particular moment and where the worker thinks they are or should be. People will often be on that seesaw of ambivalence (3.4) when they talk about possible change. In one sentence, they may be in contemplation, the next in preparation, and then a minute later back to contemplation. This is where the idea of dancing (not wrestling) comes in (see 4.10.1 for more). We need to listen carefully to the other person and respond to where they are at that moment, shifting our position in time with them as they move with their thoughts and feelings. This is very much like dancing, shifting and moving with a partner without treading on their feet!

3.9 Relapse or a Trip / Slip Up

Returning to an old behaviour is very normal. Some people will slide back one or two stages for a period and others will go right back to precontemplation. Tripping or slipping up or relapse isn't a failure – rather, it is normal, but people often believe it to be a failure. They can feel despondent and hopeless and consequently can return right back to precontemplation. But not achieving or maintaining a behaviour change immediately is very common, and it can take a number of attempts to sustain altered behaviours. Not only are relapses part of making changes but they have benefits, enabling people to identify what needs to be done differently in the future to make that change work. We have a significant role here, in animal health and welfare work, to enable people to learn from attempts to change that don't go according to plan and to continue to support their endeavours to make change. We will look at how we can do this in the chapters ahead.

It is important to remember that people can move between the stages of change quickly or slowly and when in relapse, they might go back to any of the previous stages, including precontemplation. Prochaska et al. (1994) recognised that for changes such as stopping the use of tobacco, people need to go through all or some of the stages of change a number of times until they finally succeed.

Box 3.10 Example

An example of moving through the stages of change several times was when I first started working with those with substance misuse problems in the 1990s and was involved in detoxing people from opiates. My colleagues were experienced nurses who had seen it all before. Patients went through an invariably emotionally and physically gruelling and painful detox. They came out the other side of a really tough experience and with a new life now a very real possibility. However, it was common for some to suddenly self-discharge and to go back to use the substance of their choice. When this happened, I would be disillusioned and disheartened. My wise colleagues would tell me that rather than seeing this as a failure, I should believe that the individual was one detox closer to finally being free of substances. I learnt to see that many people needed to detox a number of times before they could finally move through the different stages of change into maintenance.

When those making changes see a slip up or relapse to old behaviour as a failure they can give up as the change didn't work out on the first attempt. Our role here is, through supportive listening and questioning, to help them explore the relapse experience and what new knowledge, information and insights they now have and that can be applied in their next attempt at change. For example, many who smoke discover that they need to avoid drinking alcohol after they have stopped smoking. A drink can lower resolve, and it is easier to give into a craving or an offer of a cigarette when under the influence. When someone sees relapse as generating useful information, strategies can then be put in place for when they stop smoking in the future and so be more likely to succeed the next time.

All of this is useful to remember when working with people who are making or may make changes. We shouldn't be disheartened when someone moves back through the stages of change.

Box 3.11   Exercise

Think about changes you have made in the past. Which of these worked, and which you were able to maintain or may have even reached the termination stage for? Did each change happen immediately or did you need a few attempts at it before it stuck?

Have you returned to old unwanted behaviours, even briefly? How did you feel when that happened? What did you learn from those slip ups or relapses that could be integrated into a change next time?

3.10   Using the Stages of Change Model in Animal Welfare, Care, and Health Work

These different stages of change can be useful to help us frame our work. In human health, as well as in animal health, it is often believed that individuals need to be ready to change before we can work with them, and indeed services in human health regularly say to people, 'Come back when you are ready to change'. However, it has been shown by Prochaska et al. (1994) that even those in the precontemplation stage can be worked with and can be supported to move to contemplation, then preparation and action and so make changes.

Workers who use MI as an approach to having conversations with people about making change have been able to engage and facilitate change with those in precontemplation and contemplation stages (much of the rest of this book will describe MI as an approach in detail, but see Chapter 4 as a start). The use of MI can help people move towards being more ready to make a change through discussing and exploring their situation, experiences, and feelings. In fact, those in this precontemplation stage can be more open to discussion than we often realise (Mason 2019). It may be surprising to hear that MI can be most effective with those in precontemplation and contemplation stages. This gives all of us, working with often difficult and what can sometimes seem to be disheartening cases, the hope that change is possible. The techniques discussed in this book can equip us to help those who may have previously been seen as lost causes when the traditional approaches have been used.

The Stages of Change Model can be shared with clients, owners, and others we are working with, if appropriate, to help them identify and explore where they are with a behaviour change. If, as workers we hold in mind the Stages of Change Model it can give us ideas about specific ways to work with people depending on which stage they are in at that moment. Some of the ideas and techniques covered in the following chapters will be more helpful in some stages of change than others.

Box 3.12   Exercise

Look at the picture of the stages of change below and think about yourself and map the behaviour changes you have made and could, or might like to make, against each of the stages. This could be now or sometime in the future. What do you notice? Think about how each feels for you.

How do the stages of change help you think about those behaviours?

Now, perhaps think about those you have recently worked with, or are currently working with, in your animal health or welfare role.

Can you identify someone for each of the stages?

How do the stages of change help you think about those behaviours and that person?

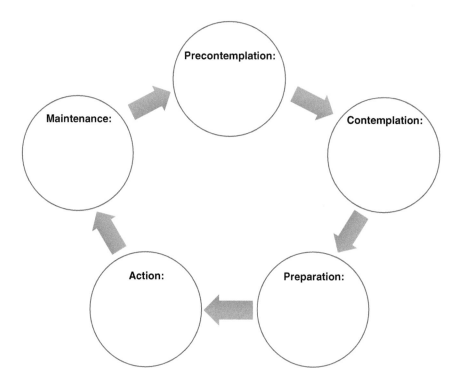

3.11   Conclusion

The Stages of Change Model was developed separately from MI, the main approach used throughout this book. However it is a useful framework for thinking about how people change and is a common model used in the field of substance misuse and other human health behaviour change.

The Stages of Change Model wasn't and isn't MI (Chapter 4); however, it came about at around the same time as Miller and Rollnick were developing their ideas for MI. Miller and Rollnick (2013) recognise that although they are two different models or theories, they are not incompatible.

The next chapter, will introduce MI as a method of supporting people to make change. The Stages of Change Model can act as a guide in using MI and other strategies. It will also support thinking about how people's beliefs, attitudes and values – driven by their individual frame of reference – will impact how they may be able to approach change for the welfare of animals.

References

Mason, P. (2019) *Health Behaviour Change: A Guide for Practitioners*. 3rd ed. Edinburgh: Elsevier Ltd.

Miller, W.R. and Rollnick, S. (2013) *Motivational Interviewing: Helping People Change*, 3rd ed. New York: Guilford Press.

Prochaska, J., Norcross, J. and DiClemente, C. (1994) *Changing for Good*. New York: Harper Collins.

Prochaska, J.O., DiClemente, C.C. and Norcross, J.C. (1992) In Search of How People Change. Applications to Addictive Behaviors. *American Psychologist*, 47, 1102–1114.

4

Motivational Interviewing

4.1 Introduction

The previous chapter introduced the stages of change, a recognised and well researched model that helps us understand how people may make behaviour changes. This chapter focuses on motivational interviewing (MI), another very well-known and evidence-based method to work with people to make change, and will outline the key ideas that underpin it. These ideas will be essential for the use of MI and for it to be effective and to lay foundations for the next chapter – active listening. As with all the chapters: feel free to come back to parts of this one at any time. All the chapters are designed to be returned to, and links are given to quickly enable the reader to review supporting elements throughout the book.

The Stages of Change Model and MI are not the same; one is a model and the other a skilled intervention. They were developed by different people; but came about at the same time and Miller and Rollnick (2013) described them as, 'kissing cousins who never married'.

Although much of this book is about or underpinned by MI, holding the Stages of Change Model in mind can be helpful. The Stages of Change Model offers a framework that can guide and give us ideas about which approaches from MI and from other interventions can be used and when they might work best. More detail about the background of MI and its originators, the psychologists Miller and Rollnick, can be found at Section 2.4.

Miller and Rollnick (2013) described MI as

> 'a collaborative conversation style for strengthening a person's own motivation and commitment to change'.

Practical Human Behaviour Change for the Health and Welfare of Animals,
First Edition. Bronwen Williams.
© 2024 John Wiley & Sons Ltd. Published 2024 by John Wiley & Sons Ltd.
Companion website: www.wiley.com/go/williams/human

This definition fits well with what has been explored in the previous chapters; about how we all have different perspectives and reasons for what we do (frame of reference, Chapter 1), and therefore, the reasons to change, or not, for each individual will be varied and very personal. The traditional methods usually used to try to get people to make change (Chapter 2) don't really work and may in fact cause more problems than they solve. At worst, the application of traditional methods can make people less likely to make changes to their behaviour.

In addition, the increasing awareness of the need for a One Health Approach globally recognises that, 'the health and well-being of people, animals, and the environment are inextricably linked' (BVA 2019). Some forward-thinking animal health and welfare organisations are changing the ways in which they work by thinking more about how owners can be supported to help their own animals. Implementing human health evidence-based interventions, such as MI, is likely to become increasingly common place over time.

MI is not a bag of tricks to manipulate people to change. Rather, it harnesses owners' own reasons for change and allows them to talk themselves into the change. As workers, it is possible to find ourselves out of sync, out of tune or on a different page to an owner. Miller and Rollnick (2023) call this in-the-moment mismatch, 'discord' (see 3.8). This chapter looks at how workers can minimise or manage discord and also how to avoid the traps workers can commonly fall into. Being cognisant of these traps allows us to avoid them more easily and consequently to have better conversations with others. More information about ambivalence is given in this chapter, including the idea of discrepancy, where a person's behaviours are opposed or in conflict with their values and beliefs.

4.2 Motivational Interviewing

Motivational interviewing (MI) is the main method used throughout this book for supporting people to make changes although others are also included. Much researched over a number of decades, MI has a solid evidence base as it has been found to have good outcomes in many areas in which human health behaviour change is required. I have transferred MI from my work and training in human mental health to animal health and welfare work, in particular, equine welfare. People in animal welfare whom I have trained in MI have used it to support those they work with to make changes, sometimes with startling results.

The term 'motivational interviewing' can, when first heard or read, lead us to think that this is an interviewing or questioning technique in which the worker is in charge, having the power in the relationship or conversation. In fact, when I first heard of it in the early 1990s, I thought it sounded like an approach taken in job interviewing. I then realised that MI is actually very different in approach and even

Miller and Rollnick (2013) themselves state that 'interviewing' may not have been the best term to use and 'motivational conversations' may have been a better name.

MI offers an alternative to the usual traditional methods (Chapter 2) to help someone make changes – in essence it is an approach for motivational conversations. It gives ideas and structures for workers to support a person to talk about their behaviour and how this fits into their world and experience. By using the skills deftly and consciously, workers can help people to generate their own ideas about what needs to change, when and how. Thus, people can move towards change themselves, increasing their intention or motivation to do so and then their commitment to those changes. It is the individual who has to persuade themself that there is a need to change.

Therefore, how we, as helpers or workers talk, but more importantly listen to others will be key in whether they are able to move towards change or not. MI is 'collaborative' (4.10.1) meaning that we work alongside the person to explore their situation and experiences, their feelings and beliefs around the behaviour. Our role in working with someone to make changes is to be a sounding board in a structured and focused way, allowing them to explore the issues of the current situation and the possibility of making a change. MI is very different to the traditional methods generally used when attempting to get others to change their behaviour. MI allows the individual to explore their situation and move towards change themselves. They talk themselves into the new behaviour.

At first, for those whose focus is animal health and care, the ideas from MI and human behaviour change can appear daunting. Workers may think that this approach is not transferable to their work, yet, the biggest issue in animal work is supporting owners and others to make changes to their behaviour for the well-being of their animals. The approach needed to work with humans is not really any different from the approach we use and advocate as part of our animal work – that animals need to be worked with in kindly and humane ways.

We need to work with humans in similar ways. Yes, an animal can be beaten and frightened in to doing what we want, but rarely, if ever, does this have good outcomes or ones that are reliable and sustainable. Forcing, coercing, or using those traditional methods for change with humans rarely has the outcomes hoped for, as discussed in Chapter 2. Working with animals requires workers to have the ability to read their subtleties, the nuances of their behaviour. A good animal person works out how to change their stance and work with the animal to achieve what is required. Examples might be when training an animal, or trying to tame one and get it to trust humans or when we aim to give treatment and care. Similarly, when working with humans, we need to understand their individual nuances with their unique beliefs and values, the reasons for their behaviours, their frame of reference.

When working well and humanely with animals, we learn when to move in or put pressure on, then when to lessen the physical or psychological pressure and when to again increase this. Miller and Rollnick (2023) state that MI is more than just being 'nice' to people; rather, it requires conversations that may be difficult or uncomfortable for the person, and sometimes, quite emotional. Working with animals is, similarly, more than just being nice to them. To help animals learn or adjust or for us to intervene for a required outcome, we have to put pressure on where it is manageable, but we must know not to apply too much pressure to the point it becomes overwhelming and unhelpful. Therefore, for those working in animal care or welfare, MI may have some significant similarities to your philosophies and how you work with animals.

The approaches, the difficulties, and some of the behaviour change issues we need to address with animal owners for the benefit of animal health and welfare are very similar to those in human health and care. Our attitudes and philosophies and values in working with the animals transfer well to working with any required human behaviour change. MI gives ideas to structure conversations with owners, but these concepts are of little use without the underpinning essential skills. However, many of the required skills may already be well used by workers from their own experiences in animal care and welfare work.

MI has almost exclusively been used, in human behaviour change, in one-to-one interventions by a therapist or worker with an individual. There are a few descriptions of MI being used in groups (Miller and Rollnick 2023) and Miller and Rollnick (2002) describe the use of MI for couples. Some of my human health and care colleagues have used MI with relatives and carers of patients, or with staff supporting people with learning disabilities. My animal welfare colleagues have similarly used MI to support their conversations with people helping or involved with an animal owner, such as a partner, parents or children, siblings, friends, or landlords. Therefore, MI is most often used in those one-to-one consultations or discussions, but it can be implemented successfully with other people around an animal owner. It can also be used, in some circumstances, with couples, families, or groups where a change is needed for the welfare of animals.

4.3 Motivational Interviewing for Animal Welfare, Care, and Health

I used MI in my own volunteer equine welfare work over several decades and taught it to human health and social care colleagues. I then started teaching animal health and welfare workers the intervention to see if it could work for them and their cases.

Recently, Dr Alison Bard, a researcher from Bristol University, has started to explore how some veterinarians have more success than others in discussing with farmers behaviour changes required for the welfare of their cattle (Bard et al. 2017). She trained some of these veterinarians in MI. She found that vets who used a 'directive style' or told their clients what to do had less success in changing what the farmers did with their cattle. Those veterinarians who were more empathic and were able to use what she described as, 'tuned and sharp listening' had better outcomes (Bard 2018). You can find videos of Dr Bard talking about her work on YouTube.

In recent years, I have worked with a UK-based international equine welfare charity which is using MI as an organisational approach (Williams et al. 2020). I trained many of their equine welfare officers and other staff, including those who took welfare calls and dealt with members of the public including those with the charity's ponies and horses on loan to them. For many of those who undertook the training there were significant changes in the ways they approached and worked with owners and others to improve the welfare of equines. These workers were already very experienced and extremely good with their people skills, yet they still found they made changes and had better outcomes using MI. In fact, often, those who had the highest levels of communication skills and were most empathic took up and used MI the best. These workers said, that by using MI they felt more positive about individual cases, their work overall, and were less stressed and exhausted by the work. They also reported being able to work with hard-to-engage groups and those who had caused multiple agencies great difficulty over time, sometimes years. These included those who hoarded animals.

4.4 How We Listen

Active listening is an essential element of supporting people to make change and is integral to the use of MI. The following chapter (Chapter 5) is devoted just to active listening, and it is recommended that you take a little time to read it as it has something for all of us, even if it is just a refresher for those who are familiar with and skilled in listening. Feel free to dip back into the active listening chapter, a number of times, as the book works through the structures and approach of MI. In fact, it is recommended that you to return to the active listening chapter as often as you see fit.

4.5 Philosophy of Motivational Interviewing – The 'Spirit of the Approach'

Miller and Rollnick (2023) are clear that MI is more than just an assortment of techniques or tricks to get people to change. They are adamant that it is not about manipulating people into doing what we want or what we think is best for them or for others, or in our case, best for the health or welfare of animals. People often sign up for my MI courses with the hope that the course will give them the ability to *make* people change. This is quite understandable as we all have difficult cases where people really need to make changes. Very often for workers, it seems obvious that owners would have better lives and their animals too, if only they just did things differently. Many of us really want people to change, with the best of intentions, and therefore are looking for that magic bullet or quick fix. This is a natural human response when working with people who need to make changes in one way or another (see the fixing reflex 2.2.8).

As in other areas of life, there is no real quick fix. The not-so-good news (or maybe exciting news if you like learning and making changes) is that using MI well requires a change in us as the worker. We will need to alter how we work and to change our own behaviour, in order to help people have the best chance of moving towards and making changes. The good news is that MI is a learnable skill or combination of skills. We need to practice and keep developing these skills. However, they will help us to help those we work with to make substantial changes, often with only short interventions required.

4.6 Discord

Miller and Rollnick (2023) identified what they called 'discord', created when difficulties occur between a worker and a client. Discord happens in all types of conversations and interactions, not just our work ones with owners who may need to make a change. You may recognise discord between you and some of the most important people in your life, those with whom you are closest! Discord is being out of tune with each other, not being on the same page. I tend to notice it as a 'scratchiness', an uncomfortable feeling or an irritation one or other person experiences or both of us do!

However, it is also possible to disagree with another person but not experience discord. Rather, discord usually comes about due to a lack of understanding or agreement about what the purpose of the conversation or discussion is, what the expectations are of each other or when there is a lack of clarity about the focus or agenda (6.6).

If there is discord we might hear an increase in sustain talk (4.9) from the individual who starts to give all the reasons why they shouldn't or couldn't change right now, and perhaps what might get worse if they made the change. We may also hear them defending their current position, or what Miller and Rollnick (2023) call, the status quo. They may say that the issue isn't really so bad or that it isn't their fault that things are as they are, or they might justify their actions or non-action.

Another way discord may become apparent is when the other person turns the focus upon us. They might say that we are not getting it, that we don't understand how it is for them, or that we lack expertise. Another sign of discord could be the owner interrupting or speaking over us or perhaps an increase in the volume or rate of their speech. Discord can be more subtle, however, as people can move to small talk or chatting, may use distractions or change the subject.

A final way that discord may be apparent is when clients or owners disengage. This may be blatant, such as not turning up, not returning calls or messages, asking to see another practitioner, or moving practices.

Miller and Rollnick say that how workers respond to discord is one of the elements that makes MI distinct from other methods and models of working with people. They suggest that discord in the conversation or relationship with the owner is the worker's responsibility to solve!

It can be helpful if we notice and use discord as a flag or indicator from the owner. They can be trying to tell us to slow down, that we are going too fast, are ahead of them in the stages of change, or are prematurely focusing on an issue or agenda that hasn't yet been discussed and agreed. For anyone, contemplating change can be concerning, worrying, or downright frightening. People often need time to draw breath, even for a moment or two, to get a sense of where they are when thinking about change. As worker, we might be getting ahead of the individual, interacting in ways that are at odds with the stage of change the owner is in at that moment. We may be focusing on what we see as the problem, or the solution, ahead of the client. This premature focus is where the worker starts to identify issues and solutions without really listening to the owner. The worker can leap to conclusions about what the agenda or focus of the conversation needs to be without asking or listening to the owner (see Chapter 6 for more on agendas).

There are some ways we might deal with discord. All is not lost if discord occurs in a conversation about behaviour and possible change. Discord will happen and inevitably there will always be times of miscalculations on our part, and misunderstandings by both worker and owner. In addition, people may enter into a discussion with us but bring feelings of discord from elsewhere. An owner, for example, may have been told by friends, people in their community, or other agencies that they need to have a discussion with us, or someone like us. It could be that a previous worker has used the traditional methods of trying to create change, and the owner brings thoughts and feelings from those encounters into the meeting with us.

Discord is different to sustain talk. Sustain talk is when someone may need to make changes, but they are experiencing ambivalence (see Chapter 8) – on the one hand, they want to consider making a change, they can see the advantages of it (change talk 4.10.2), but on the other, they have concerns about how it will be, how difficult it might be (sustain talk 4.9).

Methods to deal with discord can be:

- Recognise it. And then think about how to reduce it.
- Step back and do something different. Try dancing, not wrestling (4.10.1). Avoid arguing with the person. Try to understand where the owner is in their thinking and feeling. Acknowledge what they are saying and ask for more information about this from them. Use reflecting (see 5.16).
- Check you are both on the same page about what the issue is (or agenda, see Chapter 6) as it is easy for both worker and owner to make assumptions.
- Offer assurance that it is only they who can decide what will be done, if a change is made (known as 'personal choice and responsibility' (4.10.4). Even if we or others have to intervene because there are legal grounds, we can still emphasise the person's choices as well as being clear about ours, or other people's, roles and responsibilities.

> CLIENT: 'You are expecting me to find a whole load of money I don't have for treatment that may not work!'
>
> WORKER: 'It will be your decision how we move forward.' (personal choice and responsibility 4.10.4)

- If appropriate, simply apologise. We may have been too hasty, may have misunderstood, or got ahead of the person. Apologising and asking them to help us understand their position can be a game saver and sometimes a game changer. Apologising can, not only reduce discord, but can also alter the power dynamics within the relationship and help make it more collaborative.

> WORKER: 'I think I may not have started this conversation well. I apologise. Can we start again as I genuinely want to understand / be helpful here?'

- Affirming; identify a positive or strength of the client / owner and state it without manipulation. Affirming must be honest and accurate and can be made even if we don't agree with someone.

> WORKER: e.g. 'You have spent a lot of time thinking about this to come to your conclusion'. More about affirming can be found in the chapter on active listening (5.15).

- Shifting the focus, even temporarily, away from the particular issue that seems to be causing the discord.

> OWNER: 'Everyone keeps telling me that my dog needs more exercise and you are no different!'
>
> WORKER: 'I'm interested in what you think is possible for you. Tell me about when you first got Sandy and how things have progressed.'

Box 4.1   Exercise

Notice discord

- *Notice in conversations what happens – listen for discord in yours or others' interactions. Notice very obvious discord and also the more subtle signs of discord. A good place to start is with your own personal relationships. Spot that discord between you and another.*
- *Notice in you – Notice the feelings within you that alert you to discord.*
- *Notice in the other person – Spot how people may respond when they experience discord. It could be blatant, outright disagreement, but it may also be subtle such as dropping eye contact, changing the subject or ending the conversation abruptly.*

Reduce discord

- *Initially, start with easier conversations or less contentious subjects when there is discord or when it is likely.*
- *Use one or more of the techniques outlined to reduce discord.*
- *Notice what happens and what works for you and the other person.*
- *Can you dance rather than wrestle (4.10.1)?*

Remember, this is not about manipulating the other person or charming them, rather it is about being honest, authentic and genuinely wanting to understand and to make things easier between you.

4.7   Traps We as Workers Can Fall into

Miller and Rollnick (2013) identified a number of traps that we, as the worker or helper, can fall into early in the working relationship or in a consultation. These can all lead to the owner disengaging from the conversations that we might have with them. These traps are described below.

4.7.1   The Assessment Trap

This is common and happens when the worker takes the lead, controls the conversation from the start and uses many questions, often closed ones (5.14.1.1). The focus or agenda (Chapter 6) is set by the worker, and the owner often responds with only a few words, or just one-word replies. These replies can be centred on what the worker wants to know or what the owner thinks they want to hear. While these consultations may be short and swift, they can lack not only detail but key or important information is omitted or missed. This can be like a short and unenjoyable game of tennis with questions being served and short answers being returned. This question-and-answer dynamic can be very easy to fall into when we, in our work roles, feel stuck, under pressure, out of our depth, frustrated, or tired.

4.7.2 The Expert Trap

Here, the worker is again in control of the conversation, setting themselves as the expert (Miller and Rollnick 2023) who will dispense answers, wisdom, and advice, often using many of the traditional methods for behaviour change described earlier in Chapter 2. You may have heard yourself (as I have done many times) giving the evidence base or the latest research on an issue. We may use long words or bemusing diagnostic language.

We are probably in our work roles due to our knowledge and expertise, but the owner will also have expertise that they bring to the table. Owners are also experts as they know their animal, their own circumstances with their own experiences, beliefs, and values. We can aim for a more collaborative way of working (4.10.1) in which both the worker's and the owner's knowledge and expertise is brought to the conversation so that there are two experts, not one, involved in the discussion.

4.7.3 The Premature Focus Trap

With this trap, the worker assumes what the issue is, or believes they knows what the owner needs to do and again uses the traditional methods outlined in Chapter 2. When we prematurely focus, we get ahead of the other person (Miller and Rollnick 2013). Often, we are using strategies that work better in a different stage of change (Chapter 3) than where the owner currently is. We may prematurely focus by jumping ahead when we may well not have all the details yet, and only have some of the information needed to truly understand the owner's situation and experience. When working under pressure, especially with time constraints and high workloads it is understandable that we try to guess or just assume why people have come to us or what the problem is and what solution needs to be applied.

4.7.4 The Labelling Trap

In human health, labelling is common – patients may be referred to as 'the appendicitis' in bed five. We may describe people as alcoholics, depressives, psychotics. People are not their diagnosis – rather they are individuals who also happen to have a particular disorder or issue. Labelling occurs in general life too; parents who are strict and keen for their children to do well or achieve may be referred to as tiger parents. It is very common to hear those who struggle with clutter or have too many animals as hoarders rather than people who hoard. As a mental health nurse, I find it difficult when I hear people label others as mentally 'sick' or a psycho when they have committed a crime or a heinous act. Many people who do bad things are not mentally ill; however, we try to make sense of inexplicable human behaviour by labelling the individual as ill or mad.

When we use labels, they lead to presumptions and judgements. When others around us hear these labels, they too can then make conjectures. We lose both our objectivity and our kindness when we label others.

4.7.5 The Blame Trap

The blame trap is an easy one to fall into, especially when someone acts in ways that concern or even appall us. We wade in and put total responsibility on them for whatever we are unhappy about. I often hear professionals refer to individuals making a 'lifestyle choice' when they are in situations that agencies and workers (in both human and animal health) see as impossible to understand, to unravel or to help with. Thus, a person can be 'blamed' which frequently leads to others abandoning, not engaging or helping them.

4.7.6 The Chat Trap

Miller and Rollnick (2013) say that the chat trap happens when we make too much small talk. A brief sociable sentence or two can lubricate consultations or conversations with owners and clients, but this chat can become excessive and unhelpful. Both workers and owners may use chat to distract from difficult conversations or emotional subjects. Miller and Rollnick cited a study by Bamatter et al. (2010) that found where there were higher levels of chat in sessions, there were lower levels of motivation by clients for change.

Box 4.2   Exercise – Traps Bingo
Listen out for the traps and make a note of who fell into them (including you dear reader) and what happened. You can do this in a team meeting, while overhearing someone else having a discussion, or even while listening to the radio or watching television. We all fall into these traps, more often than we may realise. Spotting and being aware of the traps, allows us to choose to avoid them. Often, the traps are habitual; like those bad habits we all have when driving but don't really notice most of the time. Like potholes in the road that we hit when not paying enough attention or on autopilot, traps are easy to fall into but costly in the long term.

Type of trap	We fell into it	Someone else fell into it	What happened / what was the outcome?
The Assessment Trap			
The Expert Trap			
The Premature Focus Trap			
The Labelling Trap			
The Blame Trap			
The Chat Trap			

4.8   More about Ambivalence – Discrepancy

The previous chapter at 3.4 introduced ambivalence: the fluid state of thinking about moving towards a change but at the same time having a desire to keep, or sustain the status quo. Change requires effort; sometimes, it is just easier to stay with how things are. Although the status quo may be uncomfortable or perhaps worse than a possible change, it can feel easier.

To experience ambivalence, we need to have a sense of *discrepancy*. When we have values and / or goals which are at odds with our behaviour, there is a gap or a discrepancy. Clark et al. (2006) explained that this gap or discrepancy generates detail that the worker can reflect back to the individual to help amplify their reasons for change. Clark et al. (2006) say that the individual needs to have an 'appetite' for change. This appetite occurs through experiencing ambivalence which is created by a discrepancy, where the individual's current behaviour doesn't fit with their values, beliefs or view of themselves.

To help to develop discrepancy, people need support to mind, or notice, a gap. For someone to be able to make a change, they need to experience a discrepancy, or gap, between their current behaviour and their values, beliefs, or what they want for themselves. If there is no discrepancy or it is very small, there will be poor or no motivation to consider change. As the discrepancy gap gets larger, the person is more likely to consider change. However, too large a discrepancy gap can be overwhelming, resulting in feelings such as shame, significant unease, or discomfort leading to the owner backing away from change conversations. Remember, it is the owner who needs to generate this discrepancy gap. If we try to coerce them or overemphasise the gap, it is highly likely that they will back off or even disengage with us and our work with them. At the very least, we will hear an increase in sustain talk (4.9).

The worker's aim is to build that awareness of the gap and then to 'mind' it. This allows the owner to develop awareness of how the current behaviour does not fit with their view of themselves, their values and beliefs about animals, and their aspirations. Not changing now becomes disadvantageous when they consider their life situation, needs, and wants. The aim is to help increase their awareness of the costs or consequences of the current behaviour but without it becoming so overwhelming that they back away.

A certain level of discomfort will occur with discrepancy, and some is certainly needed to give energy to fuel change; but be cautious to not increase that discomfort to such a level that it is not useful or tolerable. A fine balance is required here, requiring workers to employ sharpened skills, attentive listening, and flexible approaches when working on behaviour change with owners and others.

Box 4.3   Values Card Sort Exercise (Miller and Rollnick 2013)

You might like to try this exercise.
At
https://motivationalinterviewing.org/sites/default/files/valuescardsort_0.pdf
you will find a set of values cards.
The cards each contain words describing values that are important to some peo-ple. In this activity, you will sort these cards into five different piles depending on how important each one is to you at the moment.
You can either print the pages with these cards and cut them up into separate cards or just read through and choose to write down each value under the five headings as follows.

Most Important to me	Very Important to me	Important to me	Somewhat Important to me	Not important to me

For example: Some values may not be important to you at all, and therefore, you would put those in the 'Not Important' pile.
Note: It is possible to use fewer than five categories for sorting (e.g. 'Most Important', 'Important', 'Not Important').

1) *To begin, shuffle all of the value cards except for the blank 'Other Value' cards.*
2) *Once the cards are shuffled, go ahead and sort them into the different piles based on how important each one is to you at the moment.*
3) *When you're done, if there are any other values that are important to you that are not mentioned on these cards, use these blank cards to add them.*
4) *Once all of the values are placed into the piles, pick 5–10 values in your 'Most Important' pile and rank them in order from 1 (most important) to 5 or 10 (less important).*

Alternatively, you could skip the first sorting step and just pick out and rank order the 10 values that seem most important to you. (Miller and Rollnick 2013).

Box 4.4   **Exercise Values and Beliefs**

Review the values that you hold as most important or very important and consider if any of your behaviours sit awkwardly with these? Is there a discrepancy, a gap between any of your values and behaviours? How does this feel? Do you 'mind the gap' where your beliefs and values don't quite match your behaviour?' Does this happen some of the time, often, occasionally? What do you make of this?

4.9   Working with Ambivalence Including Sustain Talk

As well as exploring a person's reasons for changing, it is important to understand their reasons for staying as they are and not changing. An individual talking about the reasons for their current behaviour, and for not changing, for staying as they are, is what Miller and Rollnick describe as *sustain* talk: a normal part of talking out loud about behaviour change. Miller and Rollnick (2013) state that sustain talk from a person isn't a problem; it just means they are voicing their feelings and beliefs. However, sustain talk could quickly become problematic depending on the worker's response to it. Sustain talk needs to be expressed and we need to accurately hear it. If we argue against sustain talk, give the person the reasons why they <u>should</u> change and use those traditional methods from Chapter 2, we stop being helpful and can even push people away from change.

It is worth noting that if sustain talk isn't there or there is little, don't go looking or digging for it. Only work with it when it is part of the owner's current experience. A lack of sustain talk can indicate that the person is, at that moment, further along the stages of change; perhaps at the preparation stage (3.5) or beyond.

Too often, in conversations with others, be it friends, relatives, or those we work with, we have a desire to get them to change by focusing on why they should / need / must change. Rarely is the individual asked about what is useful to them about their current situation.

If we think about someone using a drug such as heroin several times a day, it may seem outrageous to ask them, 'What is good or helpful to you about heroin?' thus allowing them to express sustain talk. Rarely do those who smoke cigarettes get asked about why they smoke, why it works for them. Instead, all our intuition is to push them towards where they need to be, towards a change. Yet, if we don't ask about their current situation and allow them to explore it, much of the picture is missing. Asking the person about what works for them, what is useful about the current behaviour, generates information that will be helpful to further explore their issues. It is also helps to identify discrepancy (4.8) and illuminate the ambivalence about change that can be present.

Chapter 2 looked at traditional methods of trying to promote behaviour change which includes telling the owner all the reasons for them to change, by *stealing all the best lines.* When we steal all the best lines, it means that the only position left to the owner is to voice the reasons why they <u>should</u> stay the same or the benefits of doing so. Thus, when the best lines are stolen from clients and owners, they have little option but to generate sustain talk and little, if any, change talk. I suggest that if we steal the best lines from owners, leaving no room for them to find change talk, we hole them up or concrete them into a corner of no change.

Therefore, stealing all the best lines can actually make the situation worse as change will be less likely, causing an owner to move back through the stages of change rather than forward. An animal welfare colleague who has great expertise in equine behaviour says that we get the behaviour that we reinforce with horses and other animals. I think that this works in human behaviour change too, telling the person what they need to do reinforces the current behaviour, not a change. We get the behaviour that we reinforce.

In animal welfare, an example might be when an owner has too many animals to cope with and is unable to adequately meet their needs, leading to health and welfare problems. In this case, it may well be useful to ask them about what, in the situation right now, is working for them, or what is ok about it. Therefore, we are asking about their current situation first, before the conversation moves to about what is <u>not</u> ok and then to what would be the benefits of change. This can seem counterintuitive at the start and almost as if we are condoning or encouraging current behaviours or the situation. This is not the case. Rather, we are being neutral (see 4.10.4), employing professional curiosity and working to understand their situation and experience, thoughts, beliefs values, wants, and wishes.

All change has downsides as well as benefits. Changing may be for the best, but it also takes time, effort, resources and perhaps expense too. When anyone talks about change and explores their ambivalence, there inevitably will be both sustain talk and change talk.

Never assume a person's reasons for change. For example, it may seem obvious that someone who smokes will save money if they stop. I have worked with many people who smoke but for whom cost is not an issue. Therefore, in this scenario, if we focus on finances, cost, and possible savings, our intervention is, at best, useless and at worst will ensure the person disengages from the conversation, and possibly from any chance of change.

We all experience ambivalence; it is a normal part of our everyday life, as it is for the owners and others we work with. We might decide, without much thought or planning, to go on a diet on a Monday morning (cheap change 3.4). Then, at work we find it is someone's birthday, and a favourite baked goodie has been brought it. Now we are torn between 'I am on a diet from today and it is important to me' (change talk) and 'I do so like that type of cake and just the one wouldn't hurt, diets are such a pain and they don't work well anyway and I could start my diet tomorrow' (sustain talk).

Resolving ambivalence is key to change (Miller and Rollnick 2013). Using the strategies from MI to explore and elicit the person's feelings and views of a behaviour will often support the reduction of ambivalence. Ambivalence could be viewd as a seesaw with the current behaviour on one end and changed behaviour on the other (see 3.4). Exploring ambivalence will often help the person to weigh up the good and not-so-good things about a possible change.

Using methods such as persuasion or manipulation will not help move the person towards the benefits of change. Doing this will probably prompt the person to immediately move to the other end of the balance, to give all the reasons for not changing, to engage in sustain talk, thus reducing their chance of making a change!

MI helps us explore the meaning of the behaviour for the person and what is good and not-so-good about both the existing behaviour *and* the changed behaviour. You will find a strategy in Chapter 8 (8.3) on how to support someone to do this exploration.

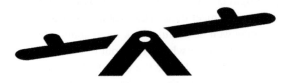

4.10   The Principles Underpinning Motivational Interviewing: Motivational Interviewing – The 'Spirit of the Approach' or Key Ideas

Miller and Rollnick (2013) describe the philosophy or 'spirit of the approach' of MI with four key ideas that underpin it as an intervention. We will look briefly at each of these. I tend to think of these as the four pillars supporting all MI work undertaken to assist people to consider making changes. Keeping these pillars in mind as we work, even with the most difficult or trickiest of conversations, can be really helpful to us, to those we work with and the conversations we have.

4.10.1   Principles Underpinning MI: Collaboration

MI requires a collaborative approach by the worker and owner working together. This fits with what the previous chapters have covered, especially the idea that change doesn't really happen when it is forced on people. Rather, change comes about when an individual is assisted to explore the issues and come to conclusions themselves. At the heart of MI is what Miller and Rollnick describe as doing 'with' a person rather than doing 'to' them.

Workers in animal health, care, or welfare, bring experience, knowledge and expertise to this collaboration, yet we don't need to have all, or perhaps any, of the answers. The owner will have their own expertise to bring to the discussion. The behaviour belongs to them. The change and how it happens will be theirs, not ours. Our role is to help them find the answers, using their own resources and expertise. Only they will know what resources for change are available to them. This might include such things as time, finances, help from others, and also their internal resources such as knowledge, skill and physical and cognitive ability.

In simpler cases, an owner will know that there is an issue and come to the worker or practitioner seeking their professional knowledge and expertise. Here, both have an easily agreed focus and possibly a shared goal. In these situations, it can be relatively easy to use MI and facilitate change. An example may be a health problem for which an animal needs regular daily treatment by the owner. The owner may be unwilling or unable to meet this treatment plan, *but* they do want their animal to be as well as possible. The worker and owner can work together on this common goal to find the best and most achievable way of ensuring treatment happens in the right way for both owner and animal.

In other cases, the professional will have different concerns, goals or outcomes in mind or know more than the owner about what is required to meet the needs of the animal. This can be more common where there are welfare concerns. Euthanasia of an animal may be an example here. The professional's focus may be the welfare of the animal and a good and pain free end to its life when quality of life is compromised. The owner's focus may be to avoid their own emotional pain of losing the animal, and perhaps on keeping the animal alive as long as possible, whatever the consequences. Here, the worker and the owner are coming from two different stances with two very different goals in mind. MI can be used here, but it will take more work by the worker, requiring an ability to be flexible through monitoring and adapting one's own behaviour (5.9) to ensure the collaborative approach is not lost due to a move to a more unhelpful traditional or 'telling' stance.

Often, however, time or welfare concerns mean workers feel impelled to focus on the outcomes needed for the well-being of the animal. This can lead to a belief that the luxury of spending some time exploring the owner's perspective is not possible. A common concern for those I am training, at the start of both human and animal health courses, is that workers just don't have the *time* to do all this listening and exploring stuff. However those who learn the skills and use them successfully report better outcomes. They find that cases take less time overall, and repeated interventions are often not required in the future. Some have commented that a little time spent now by using MI is a good investment overall.

In training, we often talk about how MI suggests a focus on the *process rather than the outcome*. In traditional approaches to changing behaviours

(Chapter 2), we tend to focus on the outcome (better diet, regular treatment or vaccinations, neutering, for example). In MI, it is useful to focus, at least initially, on the process, or the conversations needed, that allow exploration with the individual of their situation, thoughts, feelings, and experiences around behaviour change before looking at the outcomes. Yet, this idea of process rather than outcome is one of the hardest ideas to grasp, and use, especially when we are under pressure, stressed, or faced with hostility or deadlines. However, when the idea of process not outcome is held in mind it makes a big difference.

In human talking therapies, research tells us that it doesn't really matter that much which method or evidence-based approach or therapy the worker uses. The biggest indicator of a good outcome, including change, is the relationship that the worker builds with the client, and the worker's own personal style. Much of MI focuses on how to communicate with the person we are trying to help. This is one of the reasons, I think, why MI can be so successful as it enables the building of good collaborative relationships between the owner and the worker, no matter how tricky the issue might be.

Thinking back to those traditional ways of trying to get people to alter behaviours, when someone doesn't change, we tend to blame them. This can be similar to how a human might blame an animal although it is their error due to poor understanding or management. MI asks us to change as it invites us to consider how we work and what is needed to meet and help the person on their terms. Just as when we work well with an animal, our style needs to be adapted to what the owner or client needs.

Miller and Rollnick (2013) give a lovely analogy for working with people to make change. They suggest *dancing rather than wrestling* with the other person. The traditional methods to behaviour change (Chapter 2) might be likened to wrestling where we struggle and grapple with the other person to try and force them to see our point of view and to do the right thing! Dancing on the other hand is something very different. The popular UK TV show *Strictly Come Dancing* pairs professional dancers with non-professionals. The professional dancer supports their partner to the learn steps and routines. When the non-professional goes wrong in a dance routine, the professional will move with them and flexibly adapt (5.9) to support them both to get back on track. This can be almost invisible to the observer who may just see a seamless dance. MI is like this – it can seem easy and simple to the onlooker. In fact, the MI worker, like the professional dancer, is attending and concentrating on the other person, adapting to any shifts or changes of direction and then gently guiding to keep them on track with the job in hand. By using MI, workers can support, help refocus and work to the individual's strengths, emphasising their abilities and building confidence for change and development.

Box 4.5 Sitting into the Canter

I often use the analogy that MI used well can be like sitting into canter when riding a horse. If you have ever been on a horse, even for a short ride, you may well remember that feeling of tightening up and working hard to stay in the saddle. When we do that, it has the opposite effect to what is intended: we bounce about uncomfortably for both horse and rider and become even more unstable. The harder we work, the tighter muscles get, and the less effective we become. Now think about a skilled rider, perhaps a dressage rider or Western rider. They make the whole thing look effortless! They and the horse are working as one. However, there is a whole lot of work going on – subtle, tiny second-to-second changes. But the rider sits with the pace, relaxes into it, feels and goes with the horse so they work together collaboratively. MI can be similar when used well. It can look effortless and elegant but there is much work, concentration and thought going on moment to moment.

Box 4.6 Exercise

Think about work you have done with a client or owner in the last week or so. Can you identify conversations that seemed collaborative for you? What made these interactions collaborative? How did they feel to you?

Now, identify a conversation or an interaction that didn't feel or seem collaborative. What was going on there for you and for the other person? How did these affect the process (and then possibly the outcome) of the interaction?

Can you identify times when interactions have felt like wrestling and times when it has felt like dancing?

Lastly, think of a time where someone, such as a doctor or nurse or other professional, has had a collaborative conversation with you as the patient or client. How did you feel? What happened? Have you also experienced interactions or consultations or appointments which didn't feel collaborative to you? If so, what happened?

Considering these experiences, what does that mean for how you might work with owners and others?

4.10.2 Principles Underpinning MI – Evocation / Evoking

Evocation is an interesting word used to describe a core principle for the spirit of the MI approach. Synonyms of evoke include to induce, arouse, remind, conjure, call, or bring to mind. When supporting another to think about behaviour change, we are asking them to bring to mind all of the elements of their behaviour and any associated possible change.

A piece of music, a sound, or an aroma can evoke a sudden thought, feeling, or memory in us. Similarly, we can prompt people to notice, think about, and capture knowledge and information present within them and to bring it to the surface, to the here and now, to the conscious. By using evocation we can draw out of the person self-generated ideas and reasons for change or, change talk. This helps the person to be able to talk themselves into change.

You will remember that the other side of change talk is sustain talk (4.9), the reasons the person gives for where they are right now, why they might not to make a change, why change would be difficult. This gives us information about why keeping the status quo is useful and what works for them about not changing right now. We need to hear and acknowledge sustain talk but to also help the person generate change talk. Evoking that change talk is much of what MI is about.

Box 4.7   Exercise

Spend a couple of minutes listening to someone talk about change. It could be a colleague talking over a coffee about why they can't resist the chocolate biscuits or why they find it so hard to exercise after working a long day. Listen out for both sustain talk and change talk. Tune your ear in for these. Then maybe listen and notice when you also express both sustain and change talk about a change that you might make.

When you hear both sustain talk and change talk, you are witnessing the person's ambivalence about change. Be curious and hear how normal it is to vacillate between change talk and sustain talk.

See if you might be able to evoke a little more change talk from an individual through gentle listening and questioning.

Evocation sits closely alongside collaboration described above (4.10.1). It requires a different stance from the usual expert professional one that we often bring to our work with animal owners. It can be easy for us to see what the issues are, and the probable solutions – after all that is what we are in the role for! Then, we give our informed and professional assessment, guidance, direction, and advice. MI requires something very different. It asks the worker to believe that there are two experts in the conversation. The person with whom they are working very probably has at least some of the knowledge, resources, and ability within themselves to deal with the issue and therefore has the potential to make the change. This potential ability, and motivation to make a change just has to be drawn out, or evoked, from the individual.

Again, this may be similar to experiences with our own animals or those animals with which we work. We see the potential in the animals, abilities that have not yet surfaced or are not yet fully formed. We see their possibilities, and with this in mind, work to evoke the best out of them. It is similar with humans; especially when using MI, we respect and hold in mind the possibilities within the individual and work to help evoke those from within them.

In the previous chapter, we looked at the contemplation stage of change and ambivalence (3.4): when the person has both sides of the argument within them, the case for the change and the case against the change. In MI, we are working to support the individual to resolve their ambivalence and to move towards the reasons why they should make the change. We need to evoke those reasons from the person.

So, evocation is the drawing out, from the individual, using their own expertise and knowledge of their situation, the answers, the way forward, and enhancing their motivation for change.

In the active listening chapter, Socratic questioning (5.14.3) is discussed, but it is also worth mentioning briefly here. The philosopher Socrates believed individuals have the answers within them, and they just need help, or perhaps evocation, to get to the answers themselves. Socratic questioning is an enquiring style of communication which supports a person to find the answer for themselves through a serious of carefully thought out questions.

More information about Socratic questioning can be found in the next chapter on active listening.

4.10.3   Principles Underpinning MI – Compassion

Compassion is hopefully something that all animal health and welfare workers bring to their work as it is required as a fundamental attitude. We absolutely need compassion for the animals we work with. We also need it whenever possible for the humans involved with, or responsible for, those animals.

Miller and Rollnick (2013) state,

> *'Compassion is a deliberate commitment to pursue the welfare and the best interests of the other.'*

Doesn't this describe succinctly our compassion for the animals we work with? This also transfers to the humans we work with, and it will be key when using MI.

Box 4.8   Exercise

It may be worth thinking about times when the compassion we have for particular animals in cases means that it is difficult or impossible to have compassion for the owners.

Think of a case when your compassion for the animal meant it was hard to have compassion for the human involved.

> *Now bring to mind a time when you were able to be compassionate for the both the animal __and__ the human/s involved?*
>
> *Can you recall a time when you were still able to be compassionate for an owner even though you didn't like or couldn't agree with their behaviour and / or views? If so, have a think about how you did this? What helped you to do this? Did any knowledge about the individual and their experience or situation help you have compassion? What was it about you and the way you thought or behaved that allowed you to be compassionate in that difficult situation, perhaps when others might not have been?*

When we are supporting animal owners to think about behaviour change, it requires us to have compassion. Perhaps, concern for the animals may mean that we have less compassion for the owner, or lose it altogether. But, in order to use MI successfully, we need to be compassionate to the owner even when we do not agree with them or when there are significant issues.

If you find that you have no compassion available or left, and it happens to the best of us with individual cases or due to our own issues, consider if you are the right person to work with this owner right now. If there is no other option but you, then be honest and don't use MI: use other more traditional approaches. I suggest this as MI needs honesty and transparency. As previously mentioned, MI is not a psychological trick or method to get people to do what you want them to do or what you think they should do. So, if you don't feel compassion for a specific case at a particular time, it is very unlikely that MI can be effectively used.

However, the evidence from those I have taught MI to, in both human health and animal welfare, as well as from my own practice, is that through consciously using MI, it is possible to be more compassionate for the humans we work with. This can be the case even when their values, beliefs, and behaviours are at odds with ours or even when their actions are illegal, dangerous, or harmful.

It is worth mentioning here that burnout and compassion fatigue are real and recognised issues. These can be experienced by many professionals with heavy workloads and who have to work with emotions, their own and others, during the course of their work. If we are experiencing emotional exhaustion, burnout, or compassion fatigue, it is unlikely we will be able to use MI effectively. That said, using MI would appear to help in protecting workers psychologically (Williams et al. 2020).

4.10.4 Principles Underpinning MI – Acceptance

The fourth principle supporting the spirit of MI is acceptance. This means that the worker accepts the individual and the situation that they are in. This does not mean approving of, or condoning, the behaviour of the individual or even their attitudes and beliefs. Rather, it means that we accept that this is how it is for them.

In MI, the worker strives to be *neutral* by trying not to influence the decisions that the individual makes about change. It may be tempting to try and manipulate or distort what the person is saying. This can be hard when there are legal frameworks or highly emotive issues, especially when the needs and welfare of animals are a focus. When we feel, or actually have, a responsibility for an outcome, being neutral can seem impossible or inappropriate. However, it is possible to be all of these things and to be neutral as well.

Much of the spirit of the approach in MI is underpinned by the work of Carl Rogers (Miller and Rollnick 2023). Rogers was a well-known American psychologist and educator who influenced many approaches to working with people. He is known for his person-centred approach in which acceptance of the person is fundamental. Rogers believed those helping others psychologically need to allow the individual to take responsibility for themselves and their actions. In MI, we often talk about allowing the individual to have personal choice and responsibility whilst we hold a neutral position.

Allowing the person to take responsibility for themselves and their actions doesn't mean that we can say to them in what might be a traditional way,

> 'It's entirely up to you what you decide to do' or
> 'It's your choice if you change or not, but there are consequences if you don't'.

Rather, we may say,

> 'Only you can decide how or even if you make changes, no one can do that for you. But I am willing to help you think about what you might or might not do.'

Hopefully this illustrates that, by working collaboratively, demonstrating compassion and emphasising personal choice and responsibility responses can be evoked from the individual that help them think about a behaviour change.

Box 4.9   Exercise

Try using personal choice and responsibility in a conversation and see how it feels and works and what happens. It is suggested you try initially with an easier conversation – like that learning to drive analogy; try it out with a Ford Fiesta rather than a Ferrari.

> *Try different ways of saying it – use your own words. Some examples might be:*
> *Only you can decide what you need to do.*
> *It will be your choice or decision how you do this.*
> *Remember to add in some support such as 'But I will help / listen to what you want to do'*
> *'Only you can decide if and how you make changes, no one can do that for you. But I am willing to help you think about what you might or might not do.'*

Rogers referred to acceptance as unconditional positive regard. This means that the worker consciously separates their own opinions, attitudes, and beliefs and leaves these outside the working relationship to allow them to accept the person with whom they are working. This could be seen as that neutrality described above.

Unconditional positive regard aims for the worker to see the person separately from their behaviours – perhaps, just as it is possible to still love a child, friend, or family member even when we are unhappy with or aghast at their behaviour. We have all probably experienced this with animals too when they do something dreadful or destroy something important to us; we don't condone their behaviour, but we still love and accept the animal (even if we do mutter darkly about rehoming the dog, cat or equine without meaning it). This demarcation, seeing the other separately and with neutrality, is required in all good interpersonal work and is essential to MI.

4.11 How the Spirit of the Approach Transfers to Animal Health and Welfare Work

For those whose main focus is the health, care, and welfare of animals, the spirit of the approach for MI may seem somewhat irrelevant. This may all sound like ideas and philosophies that have little to do with animal work. However, I would again suggest that many of these attitudes are central to our approach to working with any animal.

Anyone who is good with animals – handling them, caring for, and treating them, as well as training and working with them – will separate the behaviour from the animal. I think good animal workers are slightly ahead of human workers here – they will not judge an animal or take it personally when they present with an unwanted behaviour. Rather, when at our best we will ask ourselves, 'what caused this behaviour?' We see the animal separate to any unwanted behaviour. Further, we try to understand why the animal needs to behave in that way. At our very best, we reflect on our own behaviour and ask, 'What did I do to provoke that response and what is it I need to do differently?'

If we have these skills and approaches with working with animals, they are exactly what is required for working with humans, especially for behaviour change. In MI we might reflect and ask ourselves, 'What did I do that provoked that response and how can I continue (if you heard change talk (4.10.2))?' 'What do I need to do differently (if you heard sustain talk (4.9), or experienced discord (3.8))?'

Carl Rogers also believed that optimism should be brought into working with people, with a hope that things can change for the better. This might be mirrored in our work with animal owners. We may need to hold hope and optimism when others such as the owner, those around them, even our colleagues and those from other agencies are unable to manage this.

4.12 Final Thoughts on This Chapter

One last point I would make here. When we work with animals who are aggressive, difficult, or resistive to our interactions with them, we often ask, 'What happened to you? What experiences caused you to behave this way?' It is the same with humans. People present with particular behaviours often due because of past or current experiences.

Thinking about the frame of reference here, some people have unhealthy or abusive experiences as children that drive how, as adults, they see the world. Some have experienced a lack of nurturing or support to develop as they might emotionally, cognitively, or socially. This doesn't necessarily mean they experienced something abusive or traumatic, simply a lack of positive care can have a big effect on humans. Again, your skills and thinking from working with animals can help. Can it be asked, as we would about an animal that presents with problematic behaviours, 'What happened to you for you to behave this way?' One equine welfare worker, after being trained in MI said that they now asked the person, 'How did you come to have this group of horses in your field?' In the past, they would not have asked but would have focused straight away on solving the welfare issue, paying no attention to the wider perspective and how the owner came to this situation.

The fact that people have their own expertise is often overlooked. We get caught up in believing that an individual is wrong and needs to do things differently. True, their ways of doing things may be misinformed, problematic, harmful, and even illegal, but they still have expertise. The expertise that they bring is about their situation, life, the issues involved and how these came about. This expertise will be key to having successful conversations about change and requires us to join collaboratively with the other person. This means neither judging or putting pressure on them to change, nor being fatalistic by giving in or agreeing with them. We need to do all of this whilst still asking them to focus on a particular issue or concerns for the benefit of animals. This may sound like a tall order, especially when working with emotive issues in which sentient creatures are involved who may be at risk of coming to, or are actually experiencing, harm. Being very mindful of our own thoughts and beliefs and responses is required. As is being able to moderate our own 'stuff', leaving it to one side for the duration of the interaction. Not an easy thing to do.

Those working in animal welfare, and my colleagues in human mental health, often find this difficult, especially when there are risks of harm and perhaps legal interventions are required. I would say that it is possible to work collaboratively, even in restrictive and risky situations in which certain outcomes are required and legal parameters may be needed, or are currently enforced. I would remind the reader of Monty Roberts who will work a horse within a tight restrictive boundary: the round pen (1.4.1). Many of the human health clients, with whom MI has been used over the years, have been 'sent' to treatment or counselling following legal orders due to substance misuse or other significant issues. I have used MI successfully many times in my mental health nursing work where my patients have been detained in hospital by law, or are under restrictions in the community, again due to legal processes.

4.13 Conclusion

This chapter has outlined the underpinning ideas and principles from MI and how these can transfer from human health work across to animal health and welfare. It has suggested that rather than these ideas being foreign or new concepts to those working with animal owners and others, a lot of existing skills and attitudes can transfer into a new way of working. Those who work with animals usually have compassion and patience in abundance. They don't blame the animal for unwanted behaviours but rather they work to understand what may have caused or causes that behaviour. Workers adjust their own behaviour to help and consciously adapt approaches to evoke the best out of the animal.

As anybody who is good with animals knows, forcing and wrestling with them to do what we want doesn't really work. Often, it causes more problems than it solves, and work can take longer with new problems generated that now also need to be resolved. It is the same when working with humans. We need to adapt our own approaches to help them. We need to dance rather than wrestle (4.10.1), to see the individual as separate from their behaviours, accept them for who they are, and be neutral (4.10.4) in our stance.

These approaches have been shown repeatedly to save time in the medium to long run, allowing workers to build better engagement and relationships with others. Working this way also has better outcomes for workers with more job satisfaction, less stress, and less complaints and difficulties for staff, managers, and employers to sort out.

Hopefully, this chapter has illustrated that those working in animal health, care and welfare already have well-developed, highly tuned attitudes and approaches that are absolutely necessary for using MI successfully. Although MI originates from, and has been widely used in, human health and care it transfers well to working with animal owners and complements workers' existing skills.

References

Bamatter, W., Carroll, K.M., Anez, L., Paris, M.J., Ball, S.A., Nich, C. et al. (2010) Informal Discussions in Substance Misuse Treatment Sessions with Spanish-speaking Clients. *Journal of Substance Abuse Treatment.* 39, 353–363.

Bard, A. (2018) AWF Research Update – Improving Dairy Cattle Welfare through Motivational Interviewing. https://www.youtube.com/watch?v=yC0uZKa0tS8 (accessed 2.4.2020)

Bard, A., Main, D., Haase, A. et al. (2017) The Future of Veterinary Communication: Partnership or Persuasion? A Qualitative Investigation of Veterinary Communication in the Pursuit of Client Behaviour Change. *PloS ONE*, 12, 3, [e0171380] https://doi.org/10.1371/jpounral.pone. 0171380.

BVA British Veterinary Association. (2019). One Health in Action. https://www.bva. co.uk/media/3145/bva_one_health_in_action_report_nov_2019.pdf

Clark, M., Walters, S., Gingerich, R. and Meltzer, M. (2006) Motivational Interviewing for Probation Officer: Tipping the Balance toward Change. *Federal Probation.* 70, 1.

Miller, W.R. and Rollnick, S. (2013). *Motivational Interviewing: Helping People Change*, 3rd ed. New York: Guilford Press.

Miller, W.R. and Rollnick, S. (2023). *Motivational Interviewing: Helping People Change and Grow*, 4th ed. New York: Guilford Press.

Williams, B., Harris, P. and Gordon, C. (2020) What is Equine Hoarding and Can 'Motivational Interviewing' Training be Implemented to Help Enable Behavioural Change in Animal Owners? *Equine Veterinary Education.* 34, 1, 29–36.

5

Active Listening

5.1 Introduction

This chapter, on active listening, is a key one. It comes around the middle of this book, and is central to what is required when working with people to make changes. Much of this may be familiar to you. However, you are encouraged to revisit this chapter as many times as you need. Like all skills, listening is one that needs conscious and continuous practice and a section (5.8) in this chapter suggests that active listening needs to be practiced in the same way as we would train for a sport.

We all like to think that we are good listeners. Many of us are, but we often mistake talking as listening. We may listen better when we are feeling good or when with people we like or with whom we feel an affinity. Listening can be harder when we are tired, stressed, short of time or we find the person we are communicating with hard to like, difficult to understand or different from ourselves.

Box 5.1 Exercise

Take a minute to think about a time recently when you didn't feel listened to. It may have been nothing significant, but you may have felt that the other person wasn't really listening – it could have been a friend, a colleague, a partner, relative, doctor, or nurse.
What happened?
How did you feel?
What did the other person do or not do that made you feel this way?
Take a minute to think about a time you have really felt listened to.
What happened?
How did you feel?
What was it that the person who listened did to help you feel that way?

Practical Human Behaviour Change for the Health and Welfare of Animals,
First Edition. Bronwen Williams.
© 2024 John Wiley & Sons Ltd. Published 2024 by John Wiley & Sons Ltd.
Companion website: www.wiley.com/go/williams/human

5.2 Active Listening

There is listening and then there is *active* listening. Often in both our home and work lives we act as if we are listening to others but it is done with only partial focus, attention, and concentration.

Much of our time is probably spent passively listening to others. There are good reasons for this. We are busy, people often tell us stuff that isn't that interesting or useful and good listening is hard work. Putting aside our own thoughts, concerns, everyday busyness and tasks to stop and really listen to someone takes effort. Often, it feels as if it will take a lot of time that we don't have. To really listen would require us to concentrate on what is being said and to use energy and attention. Yet, when we are the ones speaking and we really feel listened to, it is helpful and can be extraordinary.

How we talk and listen in social situations tends to carry over into how we listen in our professional and home lives. Think about being in a social situation, perhaps having a coffee or a drink with a friend. We take turns to speak, and as the other person is talking, we are usually semi-listening whilst thinking,

> '*Oh! I can mention my holiday plans / kids / work situation / new dog... once they stop saying their bit...*'

We politely take turns to talk and to listen, but probably, most of us are not fully hearing what is actually being said, or more importantly, the emotions, context, and subtleties. Instead, we are rehearsing and lining up what we will say just as soon as we get the opportunity to speak.

Really listening, or active listening, needs us to focus absolutely on the other person. It is not dissimilar to working with an animal, especially when trying to train them. If we begin working with an animal with our attention on something else, perhaps issues and conversations we have running in our heads, it is unlikely that we, or the animal, will get the best out of the training session. If we think about the next thing we have to do that day, or what happened earlier that day, we are not really present in the work. For a good training session, we need to be active, attentive and engaged with the animal, watching, listening, and sensing changes in them, noting nuances and tiny indicators. All other thoughts and concerns are put aside for the time being.

So it is with active listening. We need to be actively engaged, with thoughts and internal chatter shut off for the period we actively listen. This requires an openness to hearing more than just the words spoken. There is a need to also register the way things are said, changes in tone, in the speed of vocalisation, hesitations, the choice of words, repetition of particular words and any themes. Then there is what we sense is unspoken. This can be identified through noticing gaps in speech, pauses, what is being left out or what is being hinted at or implied. Then, there are the emotions we pick up, both through what is said and through non-verbal cues. Rogers and Fearson (1957) describe, 'listening for total meaning' and state,

> *'Any message a person tries to get across usually has two components: the content of the message and the feeling or attitude underlying this content'.*

Actively listening is a real skill which can be developed and improved, just like muscles can be built up and developed with correct use. It is going to be a fundamental skill for all of the MI and other ideas, structures and techniques covered in this book.

5.3   An Active 'Stance' for Active Listening

When using MI we support and help the individual to explore a behaviour change by providing structure for the discussion and a focus on specific issues or areas. There is a need for an active stance in the work and – much like working with animals – there is a purpose and an intent but with an accompanying softness and supportiveness.

5.4   Communication and How We Do It

Many people working in animal health and welfare can feel a bit daunted by some of the active listening required for behaviour change conversations, and often feel that it is not part of their professional background or skillset. However, those working in animal welfare and care are very often exceptionally skilled communicators with both animals and humans.

Supporting behaviour change in people takes skill from the worker, with continual awareness, monitoring and evaluation of what is happening with the other person and with us as the worker. You may feel that this is not your area of expertise, but again, think about the skills you have already and how they might transfer to this work. It may appear counterintuitive but, when using MI to support someone to explore a behaviour change it helps if we have confidence in our <u>not</u> knowing all the answers. It helps if we don't feel compelled to take responsibility for what the owner decides to do or not do and if we can avoid the urge to make everything all right; or we resist the fixing reflex (Miller and Rollnick 2023) (2.2.8). This often means not knowing which direction the conversation may go and what may underlie or underpin the person's behaviour and reasons for changing or not changing.

Active listening can be like feeling our way in the dark, often sensing, rather than seeing, what may be around us. Again, liken this to your work with animals. With an animal, which may be sick or we need to assess their health, we start by feeling our way. Perhaps starting by running hands over them, feeling the nuances, tensions, quality of the coat, their reactions. Then, we start to work in more specific areas, again noticing reactions that may indicate pain or discomfort or slight relaxation. We may note an area of tension or possible pain and move away from that for a little while, working more with other areas and then come back to focus again on the area of concern. Working at the animal's pace, we adapt to the feedback they give us through cues and clues. Active listening can be like this as we sense our way into the other person's world.

5.5 Non-verbal Communication

Those who work with animals may be very attuned to their non-verbal cues. Similarly, non-verbal cues are important in communication between humans and are key in active listening. Those working with animals may be ahead of the game in reading non-verbal communication; those skills may just need to transferred from understanding animals to consciously watching for non-verbal cues in humans.

You will know these but a quick reminder of some of the non-verbal methods of human communication.

Eye contact and how it is sustained or avoided. Too much or too little eye contact can make the other person uncomfortable and reduce their ability to be open about their thoughts and feelings. Too little and we may appear to not be listening. Too much can be perceived as staring and threatening. Eye contact is generally more maintained by the listener and less by those speaking. It may also differ between cultures.

Body posture. An open body posture can indicate an interest in the other person and their experiences. For example, this means not crossing our arms, or turning away. We also need to look attentive without being too intense. Slightly leaning forward can be helpful, but too much and it becomes intense and even intimidating. Too relaxed a body posture and we can look casual, unprofessional or uninterested.

Proximity to the Individual. Proximity leads on from body language. We don't need to be in a counselling-type situation with chairs drawn up facing each other for good listening. Working in animal health and welfare, often we stand alongside the owner and focus on the animal. This side-by-side stance can be ideal, less intimidating and often encourages people to share information, details, concerns, feelings and beliefs about their situation. Indeed, being aside someone can help in active listening and when having difficult conversations. Many of those I have trained, have used the techniques to support behaviour change while leaning over a farm or field gate or walking with an owner across a field.

Facial expressions. These need to be authentic but avoiding emotional extremes such as shock and disgust. We also need to look interested! We learn not to flinch at a deep, infected, and smelly wound or a badly broken limb. Similarly, we can learn to respond helpfully with our facial expressions when clients or owners give unusual information, or when we hear something that is at odds with our own knowledge, beliefs, values, or the evidence base.

Stillness and movement. Listeners moving too much or fidgeting can be unnerving to the person speaking. Also be aware, if you can, of habits such as clicking a pen or jangling loose change in a pocket. These small behaviours can be very off-putting and may stop people from talking fully to us.

Attending is a key part of active listening. Attending to the other person when listening is indicated in many ways, including eye contact, open body posture, and verbal prompts such as 'uh-huh'.

Box 5.2   Exercise

Think back to when you last had an appointment with a doctor or nurse and how they demonstrated, or not, attending to you and what you were saying. If, during your consultation they had been turned away from you, typing into their computer, and looking at on-screen notes, without any eye contact, would you have felt listened to? Inhibited in what you said? You may not have told them all that was concerning you.

Consider another scenario. You are making a purchase of an important and expensive item. If the sales person doesn't appear to be attending to you, through their non-verbal communication, you may feel not listened to, even before they say anything. Might they lose a sale because you disengage and decide to go elsewhere?

Human non-verbal communication can be immensely important when working with behaviour change as owners may, through their non-verbal communication say as much, if not more, than their spoken words. An example where non-verbal communication says more than was spoken might be when someone tell us that everything is fine but they look very sad. When there is a mismatch between verbal and non-verbal communication, we might consider reflecting this back to the speaker. An example of this might be,

'When you say everything is fine, you look very sad...'

You will find much more on reflecting back to the speaker what they have said and communicated non-verbally later in this chapter (5.16).

Box 5.3 ·Exercise

If you can bear it, ask a colleague or friend or family member if they can tell you about any (possibly annoying) habits you have when you are listening to people.

An example of this is my lovely equine dentist who has a habit of sticking her tongue out while she is concentrating and rasping teeth. This is a rather endearing and funny quirk; however, if she did this whilst I was talking about something that concerned or upset me, that quirk could impact my ability to talk to her.

5.6 A Communication Model – Thomas Gordon

A simple model that can be used to help understand communication is by Thomas Gordon, an American psychologist and colleague of Carl Rogers (4.10.4). Gordon's work centred on skills to aid communication and reduce conflict and so improve relationships at home, work, or school.

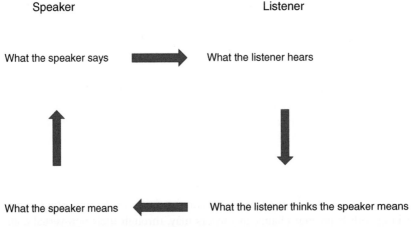

Source: Adapted from Thomas Gordon (1970)

This model of communication is simple and can help us to stop and think about how we are communicating. The first thing I like to think about are the arrows in the model. These arrows are all the areas where a message can be misconstrued or perhaps lost in translation. How we communicate at home with our nearest and dearest, often without thinking much, might illustrate this model. We, as a speaker, may say, 'Have you taken the bins out?'

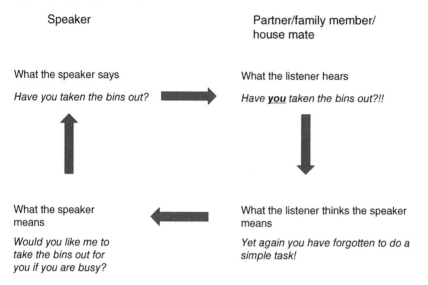

Speaker   Partner/family member/
                                                     house mate

What the speaker says   What the listener hears

Have you taken the bins out?   *Have **you** taken the bins out?!!*

What the speaker   What the listener thinks the speaker
means   means

Would you like me to   *Yet again you have forgotten to do a*
take the bins out for   *simple task!*
you if you are busy?

The example above may be a type of experience that we all recognise. It demonstrates how easy it is to misunderstand or misconstrue what is being said. Listening, and doing it well, requires an accurate understanding of not only what is spoken but also what is meant or implied.

Saying back to the speaker, or reflecting, what has been said, or what we think is being said, is key to good listening and also fundamental to MI.

Box 5.4   A Problem Shared, (*and Clarified*) Is a Problem Halved

The old saying, that a problem shared is a problem halved, can be very true. However, I would go further and suggest it isn't the sharing that reduces the problem, but rather it is the quality of the listening done by the person with whom the problem is shared. The use of active listening, especially reflecting, to allow the speaker to clarify for themselves the problem, can be very powerful. Often, that alone may be all that is needed. Not platitudes or suggestions of solutions but instead an accurate and helpful offering back of what has been said. This, when done well, allows the person to view the issue out in the open, rather than it just rattling around in their head. This allows the speaker to hear their words given back to them, to get a sense of meaning and to aid clarification of their situation. This is almost like the listener is holding up a physical mirror for the speaker to see their world reflected, which can be very powerful.

A deeper level of experience can be facilitated when the listener reflects back accurately not only what was said and half said, but also what the listener senses is unsaid. This gives the speaker a sounding board or mirror to help them to start to make sense of things themselves.

The speaker may then say, 'No, it isn't quite like that I think... rather, it is ...' When this happens, don't necessarily think that you, as listener, have got it wrong; rather, reflecting has helped the individual clarify their thoughts and feelings. Careful listening and reflecting back what has been said and implied helps not only the speaker but also the listener, by allowing confirmation that they have understood correctly.

Now, we can start to see the importance of excellent active listening, especially the reflecting back to the speaker of what has been heard. This helps to evoke, to draw out change talk (4.10.2) including the owner's reasons for any change and to allow them to talk themselves into the new behaviour. As previously described, resolving ambivalence (3.4, 4.8, 8.2) is key to behaviour change. That resolution is supported by how we, as the listener, respond to what is said and how skilfully we choose what, how and when to reflect back to the speaker.

5.7 Use of Silence

The use of silence is a key part of active listening. Not saying anything when used as a powerful listening tool may, at first, appear strange. As a listener, being silent is a deliberate, and sometimes difficult act, especially when the speaker has stopped talking. However, silence is more than just not saying anything. It is a judgement and a skill.

Allowing and holding silence in a conversation can feel uncomfortable, and we may feel pressure to fill that gap. When actively listening, and especially when using MI, silence can be used to support the speaker to consider, to gather their thoughts, to get in touch with their feelings and to think about the issues and the options available to them.

Ambivalence is a fundamental part of considering a behaviour change (4.8), so when an owner starts to weigh up staying as they are versus maybe making a change (contemplation stage 3.4) it can be hard and may have an impact upon them. The worker not rushing in and talking, but rather by holding the silence, allows the owner to explore and make sense of the situation. Doing this can really let an owner process what is going on and to experience their ambivalence.

Some people think and speak faster than others. So, with some owners, we may need to allow pauses more often if they are someone who considers their words before speaking. Others may speak faster and think out loud. We need to adjust our pace to that of the speaker. Naturally, for those who are more reflective and formulate ideas before speaking, there will be longer pauses.

Then, there are silences where people have to stop, to really think and come to terms with any realisations about changing or not changing and what that might mean for them.

Box 5.5   Importance of Silence – Example – Keith and His Shed

My good friend and colleague Keith is someone who speaks rapidly and is very open with his thoughts and feelings. In live demonstrations in our training, Keith is often the client and I the worker. He will bring a real behaviour change to the demonstration. Keith will talk at top speed and then, at points, if I am working well and making him think and consider, he will suddenly stop, look up at the ceiling, and it is evident that he is thinking. I know to wait and sometimes, wait some more. Then, he will suddenly make eye contact again and come out with something that is really relevant to his behaviour change.

I laughingly call this 'Keith going into his shed'. I liken his mind to a shed, and sometimes, he needs to retreat to it and have a rummage about in there to find the important item he is looking for, and then, he comes back out brandishing it. What is important here, is knowing when to let Keith stop, to not interrupt him and to wait in silence. If I interjected and broke that silence for him, it is probable that he would lose his place, the connections he was making, and he would come out of his 'shed' without the important idea or connection that would help him make a change.

We may be silent, actively and consciously, but we still need to show we are absolutely connected to the speaker by being attentive. Our body language, eye contact, and other non-verbal communication, perhaps a small nod or two, will be imperative.

Box 5.6   Managing Silence When We Are Uncomfortable with It

The skilful and active use of silence is hard, and like the other listening skills, especially the more specific MI skills, it needs to be practiced consciously.

One of the methods I use when I need to sit, or stay, with silence is to count seconds slowly in my head – 'one Mississippi, two Mississippi' and so on. I do this with absolute focus on, and eye contact with, the speaker. This allows me to slow down and remind myself that time is moving more slowly than I might think.

Another technique I use is to notice my breathing and slow it down, making it more regular. This helps calm me and allows me to stay with the silence, which may feel uncomfortable.

These are just some techniques I have found to work for me, you may have, or find, others that work for you. However, the more we sit with silence, when it is required, the easier it becomes.

5.8 Active Listening – Practice Like a World Class Athlete

Keith, who has co-trained MI with me for many years, says listening is like playing sport. He usually uses top tennis players as an example, picking someone like Roger Federer or Serena Williams. He will ask training groups if Federer or Williams would go and play at Wimbledon, and then the rest of the time just lie on their sofa and drink beer and think they are the best in the world at tennis. The answer from the group is always, 'No!'.

These top sports men and women work hard, very hard, to get to and stay at the top of their game. They practice, probably around six to seven hours each day. What's more, that practice isn't just a complete tennis match or a game. They break down skills into components and focus on and practice those; for example, working on particular shots such as forehand, backhand, or serve. They will have a coach who gives them feedback. When not actively practicing, they may be watching videos of their performance and that of others, including opponents, and reflecting on what worked and what didn't.

Active listening skills are essential for pretty much any work that people do when other humans are involved. Many people are naturally skilled at listening, just as top athletes come with natural advantages to underpin their abilities. However, for such an important skill as active listening, we generally invest little or no time in thinking about or practicing it. We may do a course on listening skills, or other training that include brief sections on listening, but much of the time we just assume we are good listeners without much real focus or practice – just like a tennis player who wants to be the best at their game but who doesn't get off the sofa much and doesn't really think about, or practice, their sport.

5.9 Being Responsive in the Moment or Reflexive

Using MI to support behaviour change requires workers to be present in the moment and to be reflexive. Reflexivity is the ability to shift, to move and adapt moment to moment with the person with whom we are working (note this is different to reflecting (5.16) back what has been heard in a conversation).

To help people make behaviour changes, good active listening skills are needed. Whilst not necessarily physically moving with the person, we will be adapting in tiny ways to shift where their thoughts, feelings, and beliefs take them as they consider what changes may or may not be made. To do this, we need to be there in the moment with them, just as a professional dancer would need to be with someone new to dancing (4.10.1). This takes a good deal of self-monitoring plus cognitive awareness by the worker, of both themselves and the other person. The worker will, at the same time, need to keep in mind all of the ideas, approaches, and underpinning spirit of the MI approach and any specific tools and techniques that could be used. MI can be complex, needing much conscious thought and is perhaps tricky to master, but can make our day-to-day work satisfying and rewarding.

To be this adaptive requires the worker to be 'reflexive' or to reflect-in-action and be able to think in the moment and to adapt to the other person.

5.10   Reflection-in-Action and Reflection-on-Action

Another scholar, Schön, who lived and worked around the same time as Carl Rogers and Thomas Gordon, described reflection-on-action and reflection-in-action (Schön 1983). These are two methods of self-reflection by the worker, one undertaken during action and the other, after an activity or event. Reflection-in-action means that a worker thinks, assesses, and evaluates their practice in the moment and adapts their approach during the activity. Reflection-on-action supports learning by a worker thinking about what has been done, or not done, and examining it critically to develop from it. Reflection-in-action could be illustrated by those top tennis players as they monitor and change position in the moment in response to others they are playing with, or professional dancers shifting and working with an amateur. Reflection-on-action for those top sports people could be reviewing videos of their matches. Those working with animals will use reflection-in-action every day, adapting to animals in the moment. Then, reflection-on-action is often used after the event where a worker reviews what they did or didn't do and what occurred.

Reflection-on-Action	Reflection-in-Action
Taking time to think back	Being in the moment / experiencing
Thinking about an event or an experience or our actions	Taking knowledge, including past experiences, and seeing what would 'fit' or work right now
Considering what could be done differently in the future	Thinking on our feet
	Thinking about what to do immediately / now
	Acting in the here and now

5.11 Active Listening Skills for MI

Miller and Rollnick (2013) are clear that top-quality listening skills are fundamental to the use of MI. Those of us who teach MI have found that workers who are successful with the approach tend to have, or develop, excellent active listening skills. Without these, MI just doesn't work. The tools within MI give helpful structures for conversations with people about behaviour change, but the use of these is very dependent on active listening, especially reflecting. I would suggest that you are more likely to have good outcomes with good active listening alone than if you have lots of knowledge about MI but use these methods with poor or mediocre active listening.

This is why it is suggested that you keep returning to this active listening chapter throughout your journey through the book, or whenever you need a reminder, or even when you want to think about and practice active listening skills to keep you at the top of your game. Feel free to dip in and out of this chapter whenever you think it helpful.

Box 5.7   Exercise – Spot the 'Me Next!' or a Warm Up for Active Listening

Next time you are having a conversation with a friend or colleague, notice your inner voice or internal dialogue. Can you spot your thoughts about what you will say next or how to introduce an idea or topic that you want to talk about? The 'Me next!'

Start noticing these thoughts and perhaps try putting them to one side for a minute or two and focus completely on what the other person is saying: really listen to the words, the underlying meaning, non-verbals, nuances and what hasn't been said.

What do you make of that? Is there anything you might change in how you listen?

All of the work done when using MI should be conversational in manner. This means moving away from a tick box or a standardised assessment or even an interrogation approach. Miller and Rollnick now recognise that motivational 'conversations' may have a been a better name rather than the motivational 'interviewing' chosen early on in the development of this way of working. The whole approach is about a 'style' of working, of having conversations around behaviour change with people, a 'way of being with people' (Miller and Rollnick 2023) rather than 'interviewing' them.

Changing our traditional approaches *from* passive listening and telling (Chapter 2) *to* active listening asks us, as workers, to make a behaviour change – a change in how we communicate. Making change is not easy, and it is the same with active listening as the essential underpinning skill for MI.

Those traditional approaches such as, telling, advising, and informing (in Chapter 2), are often used to try to push people into changing behaviours. We know however, that these methods generally don't work for you and I when we need to make a change, and similarly they don't tend to work for other people. Therefore, in MI, there is a move away from the worker doing most of the talking to doing more listening. This listening needs to be skilled and highly developed. When workers do talk, it is carefully thought out and focused not on themselves, but rather on the owner (using reflection-in-action 5.10). Clark et al. (2006) have a lovely way of describing how listening works in MI, 'Motivational Interviewing changes who does the talking'.

Miller and Rollnick (2013) state that MI changes who advocates for, or leads in, the change. Therefore, using MI in animal health and welfare work means it is no longer the professional or worker who is in charge of the conversation about behaviour change – it is the owner. Active listening is key for this shift in who leads the conversation.

Let's think back to the four aspects of the 'spirit of the approach' or underpinning supporting pillars of MI: collaboration (4.10.1), evocation (4.10.2), compassion (4.10.3), and acceptance (4.10.4). Active listening is key to these four aspects. Accurate active listening allows us to demonstrate *acceptance* of and *compassion* for the individual and their world. We are not necessarily agreeing with or condoning their actions, beliefs, or behaviour, but rather we are accepting the person and what they are telling us. Active listening ensures we are working in *collaboration* with the individual by exploring with them what may need to change, and allows the *evocation,* the pulling out of the owner's reasons for the current situation and for possible change.

5.12   Three Communication Styles: Direct, Follow, Guide

MI suggests three different communication styles that can be adopted in our conversations: direct, follow, and guide (Miller and Rollnick 2023). None of these are wrong; all are appropriate, depending on the issue and what the other person wants from the conversation. Use of these styles needs to be flexible, fluid and for workers to be able to switch between them from moment to moment (5.9) according to what is needed.

5.12.1 Direct

When using a direct style, we offer expertise, may give information, advice, or suggest a plan for the owner. This approach is not wrong; it just needs to be used when it is most helpful to the other person. In the different stages of change (Chapter 3), people will require diverse methods of interaction from workers. People may want guidance and information, often in the preparation stage (3.5) but sometimes in the other later stages of action and maintenance (3.6, 3.7) and at these stages a direct style can be appropriate and meet their needs. A direct style may be the most appropriate approach in certain situations too. In an emergency or where there is imminent risk, a direct style may also be appropriate. For example, in the event of a fire we would want a fire officer to direct, to tell us what we should do, how and when. If a child runs in to the road we will need to intervene swiftly and decisively and be directive in style.

I quite often liken this to those times when we are actively leading a dog or a horse – we are perhaps in front of them and in charge and they are following our instructions and directions.

5.12.2 Follow

In follow style, we use listening and understanding, giving the owner free rein to talk about their situation and problem – we follow and they take the lead, we do not offer any suggestions or answers. This can be likened to letting our dog take the lead as he goes to all the nice smells he wants to explore and the things he wants to look at. The person (or the dog!) is in charge here, and the route may be meandering and circuitous but can be interesting and sometimes illuminating.

The listener, by using a follow style, can find out how the speaker sees the issues, their perspective, and how these fit within their wider world view. Allowing them to speak, and to simply be heard can, in itself, be immensely powerful. This can be a useful style to use when there are no right answers, when the individual needs to explore their issues and wider experience. It can also be useful at the start of a conversation, a new topic or issue, and so allow the speaker to vocalise their perspective, views, and concerns.

However, if all we do is follow, to meander, it can take time and lack helpful structure. Both worker and owner may become frustrated as progress may be slow or not be forthcoming. If solely a follow style is used it may allow the person to stay stuck in one place, going round and round, or over and over their problem. Only using follow could support someone to stay in contemplation or even get stuck in a contemplation that becomes chronic (3.4).

Box 5.8   Follow Exercise

Can you think of a client or owner or even a friend who talks to you about some-thing that they might, should, ought to change but haven't been able to do? They may return many times to the subject often over a long time, repeating the same things but with no change (they may be in chronic contemplation 3.4). If you have experienced this, what type of listening do you use? Is there anything else you could do? One option could be to ask them –'what do you want from me? What can I do that would be helpful to you in this stuck situation?' Asking this can assist us to move towards guide as a style.

5.12.3   Guide

Using guide, the worker and the owner work in collaboration (4.10.1). The worker takes a more active stance in the conversation than in follow, but without using a direct style. Guiding requires careful listening to allow the owner to find their way, balanced with the provision of structure and direction from the worker. I liken this to leading a horse in hand. This works best when we are leading from the horse's shoulder; we and the horse have an understanding and a focus about what we are doing together – it is an active collaborative experience. There is a shared direction of travel. We may need to bring the horse's focus back to what we are doing together, but we are neither following by trailing after the horse wherever they decide to go, nor are we out in front, pulling the horse to where we want them.

Box 5.9   Example

Many of our colleagues have found that one of the best ways of experiment-ing with these three styles is when they are with a friend or family member who wants to talk through an issue. By being aware of direct, follow, guide, and trying them out, we may get very different responses and reactions with each style. Some colleagues find that asking the person what it is that is needed or wanted from them can be quite surprising. One of my co-trainers, Kelly, was taken aback when she asked this in a phone call with friend with a difficulty. The friend replied, 'I want you to tell me what to do'. It was then clear that the friend wanted and needed a direct style response. However, Kelly was sur-prised as she had assumed that the friend was looking for a follow or perhaps a guide type of style from her. In fact, if Kelly had used either follow or guide, her friend may have found it unhelpful and in the worst case scenario, may have discontinued the call.

Box 5.10 Exercise

Next time you are talking to a friend, notice when you are using follow, when direct, and when guide. How do these work in different situations? Could you consciously (reflection-in-action 5.10) switch from one to another? What happened if you did? Could you ask the other person what they need from you – do they want you to just listen (follow), to give advice (direct), or to help them find an answer themselves (guide)?

5.12.4 Using Follow, Direct, and Guide

During many conversations, we will need to adapt and perhaps use all three of these styles. Often when we first come across someone, we may ask an open question (5.14), such as 'tell me about your situation', 'how can I help you today?', or 'tell me what the issue seems to be'.

We then *follow* for maybe a couple of minutes as they outline the situation or issue. We may reflect (5.16) back what we have heard and ask more supplementary questions to narrow down the focus of the conversation and the information from the owner. We may well then move to *direct* if we need to give a treatment plan or information. *Guide* will be essential where we need to help the owner consider any changes they might need to make. In MI, all three styles are used, but much of the work is likely to be in guide, working with the owner in a collaborative way but with an agreed focus (or agenda, see chapter 6). Our part of the conversation, and which of the three styles to use, needs conscious consideration (reflection-in-action 5.10). Flexibly using different styles, plus the structures MI provides, will help keep both the owner and worker on track, working efficiently and with a good pace but with the worker having the ability to be adaptable, and so to dance, not wrestle (4.10.1).

Hopefully, this illustrates the need for the worker to use reflection-in-action (5.10). To be aware of subtle changes in the speaker and, as listener, make adaptions repeatedly to meet what the owner requires, allowing the owner to feel heard and the conversation to be kept focused. An example of shifting and altering styles is perhaps an emergency situation when direct may be the style that is essential but following and/or guiding can be employed by the worker once the urgency is resolved.

Remember with the follow, direct, and guide styles that if we miss the mark and use a style that is contrary to what the speaker needs or wants at that moment, the conversation, and our helpfulness, may be impaired. If Kelly, when supporting her friend in the example above, had provided a following style, she would not have given what her friend needed at that time. It is useful to consider asking the person what it is they want from us or how we can be useful to them. Why guess when we can just ask?

Now, we will take a deeper look at specific ways and skills to apply active listening when using MI, particularly the use of reflecting.

5.13 Active Listening – Specifically for MI

How can we take active listening further, use it in specific ways, to help people to explore their situation and to make changes? The following will give some ideas.

Miller and Rollnick (2023) give an aid to remember some key communication elements for MI – **OARS**

O – Open Questions
A – Affirming
R – Reflecting
S – Summarising

5.14 OARS – Open Questions

5.14.1 The Use of Questions

We are all familiar with the use of questions to obtain information, but these are often overused. Whilst questions are helpful, they need to be appropriate to the individual and fit within the overall structure of the conversation. When using MI, questions need to be mindfully formulated and used.

5.14.1.1 Closed Questions
Closed questions require one- or two-word answers, often just a yes or no. They can be useful to elicit a quick and definitive answer, but they can also close down conversations. Closed questions can also take discussions in the direction that the worker wants (direct style 5.12.1), rather than being helpful or focused on where the owner wants, or needs, to go (follow 5.12.2 or guide 5.12.3). The overuse of closed questions can be more about the worker's difficulties; we can fall into using them when we are stuck and don't know how to take the conversation forward, or if we are frustrated, tired, or feel under pressure to get things done. Closed questions can seem easier and quicker, but when overused or used inappropriately, they can cause problems for all involved.

Examples of closed questions	Examples of open questions
'Have you wormed your dog?'	'How have you taken measures to control worms in your dog?'
'Has your cat been sick?'	'What symptoms have you noticed in your cat?'
'Do you think your animal is overweight?'	'What do you see as a healthy weight for a dog like yours?'

5.14.1.2 Open Questions

When closed questions are used, people often give the answers that they think are required. Open questions from the worker allow the owner to give richer information, to expand on their perspective, experiences, and issues. Open questions are more person-centred (4.10.4); the owner volunteers their situation, thoughts and feelings rather than giving answers tailored to what they think others want to hear.

People may still give short answers. However, if we use open questions, underpinned with the qualities needed for MI, of compassion, acceptance, collaboration, and evocation (4.10–4.10.4) the speaker is very likely to feel that we are truly interested in them and what they have to say. They are less likely to think we are trying to trick or manipulate them into saying and doing what we, or others, want them to do.

However, avoid asking multiple questions before allowing the speaker to answer, for example, 'How is your dog, are you planning to neuter and has he been wormed recently?'

Another problematic questioning technique is forced answer questions where the worker gives expected answers within the question, for example, 'is vaccination something you want to do, don't want to do or are undecided about?'

5.14.2 Reflecting to Questioning Ratios

MI suggests some helpful ratios when using questions and reflecting (Miller and Rollnick 2013). These support us to consciously use questions more sparingly. This does, however, take some thought.

Box 5.11   Reflecting to Questioning Ratios
1) Ask open rather than closed questions 2) Try not to ask more than two questions in a row 3) Make two or even three reflective statements for every question used

> **Box 5.12   Exercise**
>
> *Next time you overhear a conversation, listen to the radio, watch TV, or perhaps observe a colleague doing a consultation or another piece of work, listen to the questions they use. Are they using closed? Open? Both? How many of each? What are the ratios like?*

5.14.3   Socratic Questioning

The philosopher Socrates believed that his pupils had the answers within them and just needed help to find the answers that they didn't yet know they had. Socratic questioning supports someone to find the answer themselves by a series of carefully thought out enquiries (questions) (see Chapter 14). MI is about supporting the individual to find the reasons for change themselves and to talk themselves into the change (4.2), so it fits with Socratic questioning.

Just like MI, Socratic questioning isn't about tricking or manipulating the speaker into what we think is the right answer. Rather, it is about supporting them to explore and discover for themselves: what is sometimes known as 'guided discovery'.

An example might be someone new to owning a particular animal who complains that the animal is showing behavioural issues. The client presents with a young dog causing problems, including destructive behaviour in the house and barking. The client is now looking to rehome or for a rescue to take it so that they can get a more suitable puppy. Socratic questioning could be employed to help the owner think about the situation and to come up with some answers instead of the worker telling them what might seem to be very obvious options. The questions that can be used in Socratic questioning can be found in Chapter 14 along with an example of how a conversation with the owner of the destructive dog might go when Socratic questioning is used (Chapter 14).

If you find the idea of Socratic questioning appealing and think it would fit with your way of working, also consider how you might use Socratic type open questions but alongside reflecting (see 5.16).

5.15   OARS – Affirming

A key skill for MI is 'affirming'. We can affirm another person by giving feedback about their strengths and abilities, their uniqueness and their humanness, by finding a positive. Affirming is about supporting, encouraging, and validating the individual, even if we don't necessarily agree with their behaviour or beliefs. It also allows us to give feedback about what good we see in the individual and that we recognise them as a fellow human with worth.

Affirming sits with *acceptance* of the individual and *unconditional positive regard* (4.10.4).

However, it is worth noting here that affirming is not about sugar coating conversations, flattering or manipulating an owner. Affirming needs to be genuine and authentic: if you can't find something to honestly affirm, don't make it up.

Box 5.13   Example of Affirming

Worker: Your dog is important to you, and you have tried to do everything you can to care for him.

Empathy sits with affirming. Empathy is when we genuinely try to understand the other person's world or frame of reference (Chapter 1) with their feelings, beliefs, and behaviours, even when their world view may not match ours. It is worth mentioning that empathy is very different from sympathy. Sympathy is when we focus on our feelings rather than those of the other person. Perhaps, sympathy can be quite selfish and empathy the opposite: altruistic.

One of my colleagues gave a great example of the difference between sympathy and empathy. They asked us to imagine coming across someone in dire difficulty, in deep water, at risk of drowning. The use of sympathy is like jumping in with the person and saying, 'It's cold and wet and I think I am drowning too! I know how you feel!' By doing this, we are not much use to the person.

In the same scenario, but using empathy, we stand with one foot on the water's edge, keeping ourselves secure and grounded. The other foot is just in the water, getting a sense of how it is for the other person. We offer them our hand to pull them out. In this example, we keep our own integrity and safety, whilst at the same time having some sense of where the other person is. This allows us to be helpful to them.

5.16   OARS – Reflecting

Reflecting involves the listener giving back the essence of what is being communicated by the speaker. It is important to use the speaker's own words and phrases, but these can also be combined with our own words. Reflecting is very much more than simply repeating or parroting back what the speaker has said. Generally, reflecting should not be longer than what has been said by the speaker, more often it is much shorter.

Reflecting allows the speaker to hear what they have said, given back to them, with the listener acting as a sounding board. Miller and Rollnick (2013) say that, when reflective listening is done well the speaker continues to talk, to expand on the issues and it allows them to consider and think more deeply. In addition, accurate reflecting of what has been said aids engagement and the building of a trusting relationship between worker and owner. This can happen remarkably quickly even when accurate and well-honed reflecting is all that is initially used.

In MI, we listen particularly for, and then reflect back, any self-generated positive statements about behaviour change or *change talk* (4.10.2), no matter how tenuous or hesitant it may be.

Box 5.14   An Example – Reflecting Change Talk

Owner: 'If I *did* look at changing things for the animals, it would mean a whole different way of doing things and that would take a lot of effort from me.'

Worker: 'Changing things would mean doing things differently.'

Sometimes, we can reflect back what has not been said, what we sense, or what has been hinted at by the speaker. We may also pick up and reflect back what we have noticed through the individual's non-verbal responses. An example might be an owner who says one thing but their facial expression or body language indicates something else. We might reflect back something like this, for example:

'You are confident that this is the way forward in the treatment of your animal, but I sense it worries you...'

We may detect something doesn't quite fit with what is actually being said, often through the speaker's body language or an inflection or by the tone of their voice.

Box 5.15   Example of Reflecting What Has Been Sensed

My colleague Keith, when he was paired in a practical session with a student on one of our courses, had a hunch from the student's non-verbal presentation that she was angry about the issue she had brought to discuss. Keith reflected back to the student that he sensed she was angry. She said it was not the case and continued the discussion. Keith listened some more and a little later again asked if she was angry. Again she said no. Keith waited and listened and then reflected for a third time, 'You sound angry about this'.

The student replied, 'I'm bloody furious!'

This serves as an example of reflecting, giving back what is sensed through nuances, what isn't being said or what is shown through body language. It also illustrates that, as active listeners, we sometimes have to go with our gut, using intuition, and also, that we can wait and come back to an issue again, respectfully and with curiosity.

Active listening when done well can look very easy to the outside observer, but it is in fact a skill that needs to be well practiced and honed to get to this level. This is similar to those top athletes who make what they do look fluid and easy, yet there is a great deal of work and thought behind it. Imagine a top dressage rider and how still and poised they look despite so much going on for them, their horse and within the communication between the two. Active listening, especially reflecting, is essential to MI. Whilst many of the techniques for MI can be easily learnt, if they are not underpinned by good active listening skills and the spirit of the approach, they will be of little use.

Box 5.16 Exercise

Listen to a TV or radio interview or to conversations around you and identify the questions, both open and closed, and see if you can also hear any reflecting. Listen to what happens for the person being interviewed when different methods are used.

5.16.1 Different Types of Reflecting

MI goes further as it describes specific ways of reflecting when listening to support behaviour change.

5.16.1.1 Simple Reflecting

When using simple reflecting, the listener repeats back what the speaker has said using their own words or a combination of the speaker's words with the listener's understanding of these.

This second reply above is still useful and doesn't mean all is lost – you have been given very useful information that shows how little confidence the person has right now in making any change. It gives you indicators about how to steer the conversation using some of the MI techniques covered in the coming chapters.

But, hold in mind that reflecting should be much more than just parroting back to the speaker; you need to convey something more than purely a repetition, whilst staying close to what the person actually said.

Box 5.17   Example of Simple Reflecting

OWNER: 'I don't have the money for all the treatments that are being recommended to me for my animal.'

WORKER: 'What is being recommended is too expensive for you.'

Or,

WORKER: 'The treatment options are not affordable for you.'

There is no one right way; you will know, with careful listening, what you need to reflect back. It will be important to pick up the nuances and meaning conveyed, as well as the actual words used by the speaker. Attention to all of these will help you decide what and how to reflect back. Sometimes, it can be a simple word or two that can be reflected back.

OWNER: 'I feel there is nothing I can do about the situation.'

WORKER: 'Nothing?'

OWNER: 'Well not nothing, I guess I could do some things, but they would take time and effort… like when I have tried in the past…'

Or the owner could say,

OWNER: 'No, nothing. It feels hopeless and I feel powerless to make any changes in the situation.'

5.16.1.2 Selective Reflecting

Selective reflecting is where the listener gives back some of what the person has said. Typically in MI this would be what you perceive as the essential issues for the individual (earlier in the process or stages of change) or change talk (later in the process or further on in the stages of change).

Box 5.18   Example of Selective Reflecting

As with the previous example of the owner's concerns about change / treatment (<u>earlier</u> in the process or stages of change), a discussion using selective reflection could sound like this,

OWNER: 'I don't have the money for all the treatments that are being recommended to me for my animal.'

WORKER: 'All the treatments?'

Or change talk (<u>later</u> in the process or further in the stages of change)

> OWNER: 'If I looked at what is affordable for me right now, I wonder if we could look to give some treatment...'
>
> WORKER: 'There may be some things that are affordable that you could look at...'

5.16.1.3 Complex Reflecting

Complex reflecting moves beyond simple reflecting and offers back to the speaker more than just the words they use. Miller and Rollnick liken simple and complex reflecting to an iceberg. Simple reflecting is the part of the iceberg visible above the surface of the water. Complex reflecting is the deeper, less visible, less obvious but perhaps bigger issues, feelings, beliefs, and experiences that can be sensed as present for the individual. I tend to think of these below the surface elements as the key issues, the ones that often keep the person where they are now, the reasons why change isn't possible for them or how frightening change would be. These reasons can be unspoken. For many people, they can be unspeakable. They may never have discussed them with anyone before, or they don't know how to do so. Perhaps the feelings associated with the reasons are painful, embarrassing, or shameful for them.

When we use complex reflecting, it can really help people to move within the stages of change (Chapter 3). But it requires skill and attention to detail. When we don't get it quite right, we need to realise, adapt and try other ways.

5.16.1.4 Types of Complex Reflecting

Double-sided Reflecting

Double-sided reflecting allows the listener to give back the ambivalence (3.4, 4.8) heard from the speaker. It offers the speaker the two sides of thinking about change that they have given. The *sustain talk* on the one hand and *change talk* that has been voiced on the other hand. By using double-sided reflecting we are offering back the arguments for change and those against the change that we have heard from the individual.

'On the one hand, you don't want your dog to be put to sleep, and on the other hand, you don't want him to suffer. You want him to have a good death when the time comes...'

'You are aware that treatments for your horse are going to be very expensive should you choose to use them... and... you want him to be able to keep working as well as he can for as long as is possible for him'.

Miller and Rollnick (2013) suggest the use of '*and*' is a better option than '*but*' in double-sided reflecting as it may be easier for the speaker to hear. The use of 'and' can be less dismissive of the first part of the sentence - the sustain talk which will be important to the speaker. However, Miller and Rollnick say not to worry too much about this but just be aware of it as an option.

Overstating (Amplification)

Overstating (amplification) can be helpful when a person makes a firm statement. Reflecting a statement back with a slight overstatement, or amplifying it, can establish if the person is adamant in how they feel about the issue or if there is some ambivalence (3.4, 4.8) and if this is an area for them to explore. Over statement / amplifying can also evoke change talk.

> OWNER MAKING A FIRM STATEMENT: 'No matter what, I won't have a dog put to sleep.'
>
> WORKER USING OVER STATING: 'Under no circumstances will euthanasia be an option for you with your dog.'
>
> OWNER: 'No, he will just die as naturally he should, here at home with me.' (adamant)

> or,

> OWNER: 'Well, I'm not saying never – if I absolutely had to, it might have to be an option, but the time isn't now and I'd rather he died peacefully in his sleep.' (ambivalence)

When choosing to use an overstatement, be careful that this isn't heard by the other person as sarcasm or patronising. Tone and style of delivery will be everything. I liken the use of overstating (amplification) to the use of salt in cooking. Used carelessly or in too large an amount, salt can ruin food. Used thoughtfully and in just the right amount, it can enhance and draw out flavours. Overstatement needs to be used similarly – with care and thought so it enhances the conversation and evokes change talk.

Reflecting the Gap

We can use reflecting to give back to the speaker a gap between their behaviour and their values or beliefs. We all do things that do not quite align with our beliefs and values or do not match how we see ourselves. Carefully giving this back to the speaker, in a kind and neutral manner (4.10.4), can be very uncomfortable but very helpful to them (see discrepancy 4.8).

For example, a discussion about end of life where there is possibly some discrepancy could be as follows,

> OWNER: 'I always make sure my animals don't suffer and I will take the right decision for them at the end, but I am not ready for that to happen to Freddie.'
>
> WORKER: 'A good end to an animal's life is important to you. Freddie is also very important to you and you are not ready to let him go yet.'

Remember Reflecting to Questions Ratio

Box 5.19   Reflecting to Questions Ratios

1) Ask open rather than closed questions.
2) Try not to ask more than two questions in a row.
3) Make two or even three reflective statements to every question.

Box 5.20   Exercise – Using the Reflecting to Questions Ratios

Try using more reflecting and fewer questions when you are talking to people
  Try the ratio of 1 question: 2 reflections, or even 1 question: 3 reflections.
  Notice what happens.

  Just a word of caution. Family or friends may be the easiest people to practice active listening with, but they are also the most able to spot anything that is different if it isn't very subtle. If you can increase your use of reflecting, and perhaps some of the other techniques described, and your closest family members don't notice, then you are using the skills with the required level of subtlety and skill!

Box 5.21   Top Tip for Reflecting

When we first start using more reflections in our work it is common to make them sound like questions each time, with an inflection in tone creating a verbal question mark at the end of the reflection. Miller and Rollnick suggest dropping the intonation so that reflections are delivered more as statements. However, making reflecting a little tentative can allow it to sound softer to the person we are working with. They may receive it better and then be more inclined to expand their response.

With experience and practice you may well find that reflecting back as a statement allows the speaker to confirm whether your reflection is correct or not. If you haven't quite got it right, it is not a problem as the speaker will usually clarify and give more information. It is worth experimenting with either reflecting as a statement or as a question and seeing what works for you and the person you are working with.

5.17   OARS – Summarising

Summarising is a key skill in active listening and also in MI. When people are talking about behaviours and what is important to them, a lot of information and detail is usually given. A summary, offered by the listener, identifies and brings together the speaker's important points.

Miller et al. (2008) liken an MI summary to the giving of a bouquet of flowers. The worker notes and collects key points made by the client or owner, as if they were selecting specific and important individual flowers. The worker then offers a summary, or bouquet, as a skilful presentation of the owner's own ideas and arguments around change. Miller et al. (2008) state that this can have a significant impact, as the speaker may not have heard their own reasons for change put together before.

Summaries by the worker are also useful to help keep the owner on track and to focus on the agreed topic or agenda (see Agendas, Chapter 6). It is especially beneficial after a series of open-ended questions to do a mini summary wherein the worker can emphasise certain aspects of what the person has said, especially any change talk (4.10.2) or sustain talk (4.9) that is heard or has been intimated.

5.18   Stages of Change and Active Listening

It might be useful here to remind ourselves of the stages of change (Chapter 3) and the following are some examples of what might be heard from owners in different stages of change and how we might reflect back. These are only suggestions, used to illustrate, not absolutes about how to do any of this. Remember your personal style, skills, and the relationship you have with the other person will be key: allow those to direct how *you* decide to respond.

These examples of different methods of reflecting depending on the stage of change at that moment also illustrate how people can move quickly around the stages within a single conversation, which is very normal.

Owner: *'Other people keep telling me that my dog is overweight, but I don't think there is a problem.'* [precontemplation stage (3:3)]

Worker: 'You don't think that your dog is overweight, but other people keep telling you that he is.' (simple reflecting)

Owner: *'Yes, especially my husband. He says I feed the dog too many titbits and treats...'*

Worker: 'Others tell you that feeding your dog treats impacts on his weight....' (simple reflecting)

OWNER: *'I know the dog is overweight, but he just looks so hungry all the time. I would hate to be hungry.'* [ambivalence (3.4, 4.8) and may now be in contemplation (3.4)– also starting to give emotional content and perhaps ideas about their frame of reference 1.3)]

WORKER: 'It is difficult for you to see the dog look hungry.' (simple reflecting)

or

WORKER: 'When he looks hungry, you just have to feed him...' (overstating /amplification)

OWNER: *'Yeah, I know what it is like to be hungry as a kid, and I never want any person or animal around me to feel hungry but that does mean we all are a little cuddly in our family, both humans and animals.'* (followed by laughter)

WORKER: 'Your own childhood experiences mean it is important to you that no one, including animals, goes hungry in your household.' (simple reflecting)

OWNER: *'Yeah, yeah, but you know I guess that means that we are all less healthy than we might be... I know that. But it is just so hard...'* [contemplation 3.4] (sustain talk 4.9)

WORKER: 'Hunger is not something you want anyone or any animal to feel, and you know that this might mean being less healthy...' (double-sided reflection)

OWNER: *'That's a tough one as I want us all to be well and healthy, but not hungry. I just don't know how to balance the two!'*

WORKER: 'You have your family's and your animal's best interests at heart...' (simple reflecting) (affirming 5.15)

OWNER: *'Yeah... but really... am I doing the best thing...?'* [contemplation 3.4]

WORKER: ....(sits with, and uses silence 5.7) (waits)

OWNER: *'I'm wondering which is worse now... ill health or being a tiny bit hungry... I guess this is something I probably need to look at* [contemplation 3.4] *... It's my responsibility to look after us all and only I can change what I do...'*

WORKER: 'It will be up to you to decide what you do...' (simple reflecting and also emphasising personal choice and responsibility 4.10.4)

OWNER: *'Yeah, but I sure could do with some help with this!'* [contemplation (3.4) moving to preparation (3.5)]

WORKER: 'Who might be able to help you?' (open question)

OWNER: *'Well, I might start with you here at the veterinary surgery. Maybe you can help me identify what is ok and what isn't ok to feed the dog and also when?'* [preparation (3.5)]

WORKER: 'You are wondering if one way might be for us to work with you... We can certainly do that...' (simple refection of change talk plus information)

OWNER: *'That would be really helpful, but you know this isn't going to be easy for me.'* (slight move back to contemplation and demonstrating ambivalence)

WORKER: 'Let me see if I have got where we are at so far...' (starting a summary 5.17) 'Other people have been telling you that your dog needs to have a different diet. On the one hand, you would like to be able to do that for him and on the other hand, you don't want him to feel hungry.' (double-sided reflecting in the summary) 'You would like some help to look at possible ways of changing his diet and one way would be to see what help and ideas we at the surgery here can offer. Would you like me to give you some information about what we offer around diet and weight?' (offering information if the owner would like it 9.7)

5.19 Conclusion

It is not by accident that this chapter is around the centre of the book. It is also the longest chapter, again not by accident. Active listening is central to helping people change behaviours, especially when using motivational interviewing. Even if you don't use any of the other ideas in the rest of the book but only increase how much you actively listen and how you do it, your conversations and consultations are likely to be different.

As you work through the book, especially the following chapters, it may help to keep this chapter in mind and to keep returning to it to refresh your ideas.

Those who we teach, tell us in the training room that this active listening is hard, and tiring. But then they come back to a following session and tell us that a lot changed when they listened differently.

This book asks <u>you</u> to make changes to what you do and how you listen to other people when helping them to make changes. With practice, active listening gets easier and can become a core skill we can use every day and in most situations. Try practicing active listening and working at it just as a world class athlete would prepare for the Olympics.

References

Clark, M., Walters, S., Gingerich, R. and Meltzer, M. (2006) Motivational Interviewing for Probation Officer: Tipping the Balance Toward Change. *Federal Probation.* 70, 1: 38

Gordon, T. (1970) *Parent Effectiveness Training*. New York: Wyden.

Rogers, C. and Farson, R. (1957) Active listening Excerpt. Available from Gordon Training International. https://www.gordontraining.com/wp-content/uploads/Active_Listening.pdf

Miller, W.R. and Rollnick, S. (2013). *Motivational Interviewing: Helping People Change*, 3rd ed. New York: Guilford Press.

Miller, W.R. and Rollnick, S. (2023). *Motivational Interviewing: Helping People Change and Grow,* 4th ed. New York: Guilford Press.

Miller, W. R., Rollnick, S, and Butler, C. C. (2008) *Motivational Interviewing in Health Care: Helping Patients Change Behavior.* New York: The Guilford Press.

Schön, D.A. (1983) *The Reflective Practitioner: How Professionals Think in Action.* USA: Basic Books Inc.

Recommended

Columbus K & Samaritans. (2021) *How to Listen. Tools for Opening Up Conversations When it Matters Most.* London: Kyle Books.

6

Finding Focus and Setting the Agenda

6.1 Introduction

The previous chapters have described how people view the world with their individual frame of reference which underpins and supports attitudes, beliefs, and behaviours. We have looked at a model for how people make changes, the Stages of Change Model which is also known as the 'Transtheoretical Model'. Then motivational interviewing (MI) was covered in Chapter 4 and how it might be applied in animal health, care, and welfare work and then in Chapter 5 the all-important active listening.

This chapter will start to put these ideas together, and in the coming chapters specific MI techniques are described that can be used to support people to make changes for the well-being of their animals. The starting point for any behaviour change work is how we first come in contact or engage with an owner, and what the agenda or focus is of the conversations that we need to have with them.

This chapter will start to look at how we might work with people who may need to make one change, several, or many changes and the key techniques that will help us to help them. You might want to revisit parts of earlier chapters just to build and layer your understanding and learning; the book is designed to help you do that and with signposts back to parts which may be useful to you at certain points.

6.2 Contact and Engagement

Let's begin by thinking about the start of the journey we might have with an individual. Depending on where you work, in animal health, care, or welfare, people will present to you or you may need to go and find them. Some will be pleased to

Practical Human Behaviour Change for the Health and Welfare of Animals,
First Edition. Bronwen Williams.
© 2024 John Wiley & Sons Ltd. Published 2024 by John Wiley & Sons Ltd.
Companion website: www.wiley.com/go/williams/human

see you and others not. Our roles might be voluntary, paid, self-employed, specialist, or generic. We may work for, or represent a company or organisation. We may be employed by government, local authorities, charities, or some other agency. Some of us will work for animal organisations and others for environmental health, social care, law enforcement, or other human-focused organisations. Who we are, our roles, and the employers and professions we represent, as well as the reasons for our contact, will bring an immediate dynamic to the relationship with the owner.

That dynamic will be further influenced by whether we are encountering someone for the first time or if we have known them for many years. They may come looking for some help, advice, or something else, which we may be able, or not, to give. We may be purveyors of unwelcome or upsetting news, or we could be approaching the owner as there is a welfare or other issue and consequently they may not be at all pleased to see us. There may be a requirement for the worker to undertake organisational objectives by seeking out and working with certain people or groups to change behaviour where their animals are concerned. For some agencies and charities, this could be issues such as vaccination, neutering and castration, or changing traditional handling or harnessing practices.

Most of us would probably be unhappy if someone contacted us to say that there were issues or concerns about animals we own or have responsibility for. Our own individual *frame of reference* (Chapter 1), may drive how we respond to and view this probably unwanted contact. It is possible, however, that some people are relieved that someone has become involved. They might be overwhelmed and know they need support but have been unable to get it or didn't know how or who to ask for help. Every case and every owner is different, with diverse circumstances and backstories and each individual has their own unique frame of reference.

Whether animal owners voluntarily seek out advice, support or treatment for animals from others, and if they then accept the offered assistance, advice, guidance and direction, will very much depend upon that individual's frame of reference.

Therefore, those encountered when we are working, or perhaps volunteering, will have unique, and sometimes not very obvious, motivations for their responses to us. This means workers have to be incredibly flexible in their approach. No standard style or response will work with everyone. We will need to adapt and respond moment to moment, using reflection-in-action (5.10) in response to the animal owner we are working with. MI gives a framework to do that with particular tools and techniques that can help.

Behaviour change and the evidence around it can seem overwhelming and complicated. Very probably all we want is a simple quick fix to get the best outcome for the animals. However, as you will very probably well know, humans and their situations are complex. Therefore, our methods of responding, intervening, and helping need to be adaptive and responsive to those complexities.

6.3 Agendas in Animal Welfare

In welfare work, and in regulation or the enforcement of laws, involvement with an animal owner usually comes about due to someone identifying and reporting a problem. Something needs to change for the welfare of an animal or animals. Reports can come from a neighbour, other people in the community, another human or animal agency, or environmental or law enforcement. Our contact may come about as part of our employing organisation's programme to improve the welfare of certain groups of animals. There may be detailed reports giving an idea about what to expect, or minimal information so what we are going to is unknown. Reports may be anonymous and sometimes, not uncommonly, reports of animal welfare issues can be malicious and driven by other conflicts. For some workers a routine inspection or check leads to an issue being identified. All of these scenarios require excellent people skills, the ability to navigate the unexpected and to help people consider behaviour change. MI can be used in all of these cases and roles.

Another issue with which MI can and has been successfully used, is when working with those who report welfare concerns. Some reporters have unrealistic or high expectations and demands. When unsatisfied, they may make threats that could impact upon an organisation's reputation. Some welfare reporters make continual contact and reports, becoming vexatious. A few reporters become well known to those taking welfare calls and sometimes to the workers tasked with investigating these reports. In my behaviour change training with animal welfare agencies, the techniques discussed in this book have successfully been used by office staff who take these type of calls and have to deal sometimes with vexatious reporting, as well as by the other workers who may also have to deal with them.

As outlined above, animal welfare work brings a wide range of different agendas from many people. In welfare calls, the reporter's agenda is usually that they want the welfare agency 'to do something', whether that be to improve the welfare of the animals involved or for other reasons driven by their desire for certain outcomes. The agenda of the welfare organisation involved may be to take and investigate reports thoroughly and promptly within the resources they have available and the legal processes for the country in which they work, while maintaining their reputation and support from those that provide funding. The welfare worker's agenda may be to get an accurate assessment done, to see if there is an issue, and to come up with a plan for improving conditions for the animals involved. The worker may also be under pressure from a high caseload, documentation, time, travelling distance, weather, environmental issues and perhaps their own personal circumstances that day or week. If other agencies are involved, they too will have their own agendas: often these are to hand over to someone else, especially if the issue is not one that they have expertise in, or the resources for. This is very common in welfare cases that require multi-agency input from both human and animal welfare organisations. Best outcomes are usually achieved in these cases when organisations all work together despite having different areas of focus, approaches and expertise, but sadly good multi-agency working can be the exception rather than the norm.

Then, for the person who owns or is responsible for the animal or animals that have been reported, their agenda is probably going to be very different from all of the others mentioned above. There may also be family and friends of the owner and other social contacts who also have their own agendas. Then there may be human health or welfare concerns or issues causing others with very different agendas to be involved, including environmental agencies, law enforcement, and others, including human health and social care.

6.4 Agendas in Animal Health and Care

For those working in animal health and care roles, again there are different agendas. The owner can present an animal and expect answers, perhaps not the ones you need to give them. They may not want, or be able to afford, the required investigations needed for you to give them an answer. They may want treatment without expense. They may have realistic or unrealistic expectations. As worker, you have a responsibility to the animal but also to the owner as your client, and very probably, you also have a responsibility to your employer as well as your professional regulating body.

So, before we even start looking at the behaviour change interventions that we might employ as animal workers, there may possibly be a large number of vastly different agendas all driven by diverse responsibilities, expectations, and even views of the world or frames of reference.

6.5 Using MI for Engagement and Rapport Building

Readers of this book are likely be highly able and skilled in building rapport with those they work with. However, any of us can, at times, lose or fail to keep engagement with some people.

MI can support both rapport building and engagement, including with those who are reticent or cannot see the reason for working with us. People who have been reported by others for animal welfare concerns can be very different to engage with than those who willingly seek help and treatment from professionals.

One of the most useful methods of quickly building rapport is through active listening (Chapter 5). No matter how angry or distressed someone is, if they feel listened to and really heard, they are more likely to engage. Skilful listening and the demonstration of the worker's understanding of the owner's views and situation will be invaluable.

The idea of a 'neutral' stance (Miller and Rollnick 2023) (4.10.4) by the worker can be useful here. We don't have to agree or condone the owner's actions or their beliefs and behaviour, but we can show a willingness to understand without condemning them. This can set a helpful dynamic for the rest of the relationship that will follow.

Chapter 3 looked at the Stages of Change or Transtheoretical Model and highlighted that it isn't only those who are ready and willing who can be worked with to make a change. Those who are in precontemplation (3.3) and contemplation (3.4) stages can be helped, especially with the use of MI, to look at behaviour changes they could or might make. Workers commonly feel that it is hopeless or useless to work with people when the individual can see no reason to change their current behaviour. However, we know from evidence that using the approaches outlined in this book can help those in precontemplation and contemplation engage and make changes, as well as those in the later stages of change of preparation (3.5) and action (3.6).

6.6 Agendas: Shared Agendas, Complimentary Agendas, or Opposing Agendas?

Agendas are different from goals. Goals are outcomes that might be achieved. Agendas are what we (both animal owner and worker) agree to focus on. Neutrality (4.10.4) from the worker is essential here as it is very easy to attempt to focus or push the person to identify behaviour change goals well before they are ready. Worse still is the use of those traditional methods (Chapter 2) where goals are set for them by the worker or others. Think again of the Stages of Change Model (Chapter 3) here. Goals may be appropriate to consider and set in the preparation (3.5) stage but not in the precontemplation (3.3) stage.

When we enter into a conversation with an owner about their animal or animals, an agenda is immediately being generated. As workers, there will be specific areas we are looking to discuss. The owner may have a similar agenda to ours if they are concerned about their animal and want the best for it, if they are looking for advice, guidance, diagnosis, or treatment. Some may come asking for information or perhaps an opinion or confirmation of what they already know, for example, that an animal is nearing the end of life. Some owners may be hoping against all probabilities that they will receive news that all is well. In all of these situations, apart perhaps from the less common but happy outcome of being told there is nothing wrong and all is well (and even in this case an owner may need help not to worry so much!), the owner will need to make some changes.

Medication may need to be introduced and administered, the animal may need to return for further tests, or the owner to take the animal to a specialist. It could be, as is common in the UK, that changes are required to how much or what owners feed their animals. Therefore, even in these relatively straightforward consultations or conversations with owners, there is likely to be some behaviour change required from the owner.

In cases in which there are welfare issues, the agendas of worker and owner are likely to be further apart, or could even be at odds with each other. In welfare work, where workers may be sent to visit due to a report or concern, the owner's agenda is probably to get rid of the worker as soon as possible. That said, there are some cases in which people are just overwhelmed, have been unable or unwilling to seek help, and are relived when someone arrives to discuss the situation.

Those who report welfare concerns will also have their own agenda, usually that they want something done. There may be a welfare issue with the case they report, but also, as people often have different opinions and understanding of how animals should and can be kept, there may be no welfare issue. An extra dynamic is when a reporter is also a supporter, or volunteer, for that same organisation and this becomes more complicated and difficult when it is a smaller, more local charity or agency.

The owner's frame of reference (Chapter 1) will also have an impact on how they seek and accept assistance and help or how they respond when a worker makes contact. Anyone reporting animal issues and welfare will also bring their own frame of reference to the mix, as will the worker. Even the organisation workers are employed by or volunteer for will have its own philosophy, values and underlying ways of seeing the world.

In Chapter 4, *process not outcome* was introduced (4.10.1). Concentrating on the process rather than rushing immediately to what outcomes (or goals) could be sought, worked towards or obtained is important. It is useful to hold in mind how we might focus on the process rather than the outcome by initially identifying the agenda for the discussion and then looking at goals (outcome) later when appropriate.

6.7 Matching / Mismatched Aspirations and Agendas

The matrix overleaf is adapted from the work by Miller and Rollnick (2013). It helps us think about where we as workers and the client or owner are and how we can create and agree a collaborative focus to our conversations.

Box A is fairly straightforward at first glance. The owner has the same aspiration as the worker and it is likely that they will be fairly open to agreeing and working on a shared agenda. Therefore, it may be possible for them to move to setting goals quickly. They may well be in the preparation (3.5) or even action (3.6) or maintenance (3.7) stages. However, people and change can be complex! It is possible for people's circumstances to change and for an increase in ambivalence

(3.4, 4.8) at any stage. This can happen if there have been changes in the owner's circumstances since we last saw them, or if they feel we have moved to a communication style that is mismatched with theirs. Perhaps we are using a directing style (5.12.1) when they want guiding (5.12.3) at that moment, or guiding when they just want information and a more directing style.

Box B is the position that workers commonly find the most frustrating, difficult, and sometimes hopeless in their practice with clients and owners. However, there is good news. It is here, for these interactions, that MI is designed as it originated and has been used with great success in the human addictions field and other problematic health behaviours. This box highlights how a person in precontemplation (3.3) or contemplation (3.4) stages of change may have high levels of ambivalence (3.4, 4.8). Remember, MI can work best with people in these two first stages of the Stages of Change Model (3.10).

Box C. In this area, there very probably isn't a role for the worker or perhaps their organisation. However, it may be an opportunity to signpost the client or owner to an agency or a resource that might meet their needs. To do this, you might want to read the ideas around giving information to people using a simple framework from MI which can be found in Chapter 9 (9.8). We might use MI techniques very briefly to support owners to access other help or options.

However, there may be an opportunity in Box C to use MI when someone is reporting a welfare concern when there either isn't an issue or it is not the role of the worker's organisation to deal with it. This can be a tricky area which needs sensitive handling as reporters can become vexatious, taking up a lot of time and energy for call handlers and others. Reporters can also contact multiple agencies, causing further precious resources to be used and sometimes generating misunderstandings. These types of reporters can also present a risk to the organisation's reputation if they broadcast their dissatisfaction to others, especially via social media. While MI is *not* about manipulating people to get what we want, it *can* be used to deescalate difficult situations and manage inappropriate expectations. These reports can be hard for those having to handle them but those who use MI in animal welfare charities describe being less impacted by these calls and interactions.

Box D. In this box, there is no role for the worker and no issue for the client or owner. At first glance, it would appear that this box is not worth comment; however, as identified by my colleague Keith Noble, sometimes we can hold onto or keep clients or owners when we don't need to. We may have supported them through difficult situations and through significant changes. We can keep the contact going when it may not be needed, just in case they slip back or something changes.

This is different to appropriate ongoing or periodic contact to support people who have made changes and to ensure they are on track when in the maintenance stage of change (see Chapter 12) – this is especially indicated in hoarding cases. However, if that is the case, then this intervention would be in Box A and agreed by both parties.

It is worth thinking about Box D when we might be tempted to keep in contact with an owner as we get something out of the interaction. It may be that we like the person, and it feels good to see or speak to them. They may offer us respite and a distraction from the rest of our heavier and difficult workload, cases, and consultations. We need to be open and honest with ourselves about why we might want to continue to work with someone when it is no longer indicated. I would suggest when we move to box D, it is about us and it is not about the client or owner or the welfare of their animals. Rather it is something different, it is about meeting our own needs. You will remember that MI and working with behaviour change is more than just being nice to someone (4.2), and there is a risk, in Box D, that this is what we are doing, being nice, and for our own reasons. This can happen to anyone, but when it occurs, perhaps we need to think about where to get support and help to continue the other work that is challenging, difficult and impacts upon us professionally and personally. Some animal workers are starting to use reflective practice; formally talking to another colleague to reflect on their work and experiences. These issues are useful to take to and discuss in reflective practice.

		Is this agenda a current wish / objective for the owner?	Is this agenda a current wish / objective for the owner?
		Yes	No
Is this **your** hope or objective for the owner or for their animals' welfare?	Yes	**Box A** The owner and the worker are matched in their aspirations, so it is easy to agree on the focus of the work and agenda and client is probably in preparation / action/ maintenance stages. MI and other methods of support and help can be used here.	**Box B** What MI was originally designed for. The owner is ambivalent about change and likely to be in precontemplation or contemplation stages. We can work here using MI.
Is this **your** hope or objective for the owner or for their animals' welfare?	No	**Box C** There isn't a role for the worker here or it isn't what their organisation is commissioning or requires. Possibly look to signpost elsewhere. A welfare reporter may be in this area though, and here MI could be briefly used to help a reporter understand why action is not required or appropriate.	**Box D** There is not a role here for the worker. Are we visiting or holding on to a case, a client or owner when we don't need to. This model can help us think about where we should be working.

Adapted from Miller and Rollnick (2013)

6.8   Working with Other Agencies or Other Workers

Another issue to consider is when we are co-working a case or undertaking a visit with a colleague or with a fellow professional or practitioner from a different agency to ours.

When animal workers undertake joint consulting, or visiting, to support behaviour change in an owner, it is very common for there to be a mismatch between the two workers' objectives and style of working. This is especially problematic if one person is using an MI approach and the other, traditional approaches (see Chapter 2) to promote behaviour change.

When co-working or joint visiting, it is useful for a clear discussion to occur between the workers before meeting the client or owner. Deciding who will do what is important, as well as understanding individual working styles and approach. Agreeing that one will take the lead and, if the colleague is unaware of MI, an explanation of the approach can be essential and can help mitigate difficulties. Many workers have described engagement with an owner being damaged, sometimes irreparably, by interventions (usually traditional) by another worker just as the individual was starting to engage, discuss the issues and explore their ambivalence.

6.9   Focusing the Discussion: Agendas Not Goals

A key starting point in behaviour change, after rapport building and engagement with an owner, is identifying the focus for the discussions, or pinpointing an agenda. As we can see above, agendas can be many and complex. Focusing and identifying a shared agenda is key for behaviour change. If we don't do this, are not transparent and acknowledge our agenda and don't explore the agenda of the animal owner, then worker and owner are immediately pulling in different directions, and collaborative working (4.10.1) is going to be very difficult.

A very simple way of being transparent and starting the conversation around the agenda is by asking the owner something like, 'What is it that you need from me?' or 'Tell me what might help you' or 'What is it that you want or need me to know?'.

Even if we get the answer,

> *'I want you to go away and leave me alone, there is nothing wrong with my animals',*

this allows us to at least start a conversation that is honest from both parties and gives something to work with. In some difficult animal health and welfare work, the owner actually engaging in a discussion with us may be a behaviour change in itself, especially if the individual had not previously engaged or has had difficulties in working with other agencies.

Having a focus, being clear about what specifically both the worker and owner are talking about, is going to be essential, even if they don't agree with each other in other ways. Agreeing what the agenda is, what it is that is being discussed, and being as specific as possible is important. If we say to an owner that we are concerned about their animal's health, this is very broad subject area and consequently it will be very difficult to use an MI approach. If more specifics are identified, for example, the animal's weight or condition, it allows owner and worker to both be clear about what it is they are discussing. Even with the owner who does not want a worker to be present, there can be perhaps a shared agenda; both have the animals at the centre of their different views, or both want the situation resolved and the worker on their way! This then can be the start of the shared focus or agenda.

Time spent on exploring and identifying the agenda is never wasted. Repeatedly in the work I and others have done, exploration and clarification of the agenda is central to enable the owner, often for the first time, to really think about the issues. Spending time establishing the agenda, be it a matter of minutes or longer, has been found to be time very well invested. Sometimes, just exploring the agenda, what the key issues or problems are, can be enough for an owner to move towards behaviour change with little further help required from the worker. Using a little time to identify the agenda is essential to productive conversations and outcomes, plus it saves time in the long run.

When talking to human health and social care staff or to animal health workers about individual cases, I generally ask them what the person or owner's agenda is. Workers often say, '*I think the agenda is...*' or '*I think their agenda is...*' or '*I believe the agenda is...*'. This indicates that the agenda isn't explicit or agreed, suggesting that this needs to be returned to and clarified by the worker with the owner. It is easy to assume, without clarifying, what an owner's agenda is and this frequently leads to difficulties.

Box 6.1   Exercise – Reflecting on Agendas

Choose a case that has been difficult today, this week, or this month, one that has stuck with you, been troublesome, or which you keep thinking about. Or a case in which you felt uneasy, angry or cross, frustrated, or irritated.

Now ask yourself, what was my agenda with this case?

And what was the other person's agenda? Do you really know this? Was it explicit? Did you find it out? Did you really clarify what it was with the other person? Did you agree the focus or agenda?

Or... do you find yourself using 'I think their agenda was...' or 'obviously their agenda would have been...'

This may highlight that it is easy to assume an agenda without really checking it out with an owner and making it explicit.

Even when there is a single clear agenda, there are often other connecting, overlapping issues. For example, take the companion dog that is overweight. The main agenda, for both owner and worker, may be for the animal to lose weight and therefore to be healthier and happier. However, the behaviour changes that will be required of the owner may be more complex. Changing the dog's diet may be required. Ensuring more exercise may be another needed behaviour change but, for example, if the owner is working long hours, has other caring responsibilities at home, or is physically disabled themselves, this becomes more difficult. Other required behaviours may include changing the dog's access to other food, including that of other pets, and resisting the temptation to give treats and titbits. Change is often complex with numerous elements.

6.10 A Word about Having a Chat

General pleasantries and chatting can be very human methods of engagement and rapport building, especially in social settings. However, they can be easily overused by both workers and owners. Miller and Rollnick describe the chat trap (4.7.6) that we can fall into as workers, and chatting is useful to consider again here. Owners may use chatting to avoid difficult conversations or topics they don't want to face. Embarrassment and shame may be masked by superficial niceties. Workers can use general chat to engage or relax the owner. Sometimes, we use chatting to avoid tricky subjects, when we don't want to upset someone, when we feel that an owner's reaction will be awkward or difficult to manage, or we don't want to embarrass them.

Pleasantries can definitely help human interactions, but they need to be very brief. Any more than a short sentence or two and they stop being helpful and can become obstructive and even problematic. Too much chat and the real reason for, or focus of, the conversation is likely to be lost, as well as time. Owners can be confused, suspicious, and frustrated if they don't understand what the point of the conversation, visit, or consultation is. Similar to workers, owners often have their own time pressures and may be keen to move on. Owners will see through general chat and it can result in reduced engagement, discord, (3.8, 4.6) and often in welfare cases, anger and hostility.

Therefore, we need to bring warmth in interactions with owners but limit general chat significantly. This is not about being cold and brusque in conversations; rather it is about bringing friendliness and kindness but into work and discussions that are focused.

6.11   Move from Multiple or Complex Agendas to Specific Agendas

Some owners will have multiple agendas, or workers may identify a number of issues of concern. While acknowledging that these may be inter-related, we need to try and identify one agenda or behaviour change on which to initially focus. Sometimes, this can be identified by the owner, especially where there are no urgent issues to be addressed. However, owners can often choose small changes to focus upon, especially in welfare cases, rather than the ones that we and others would really like them to change. Whenever possible, going with the owner's identified agenda can allow them to have control over what might change. This also allows smaller and simpler changes at first to help the build their confidence that changes can be possible for them (see 7.10–7.14 and 9.4). If more urgent issues need to be addressed, then the worker will need to skilfully negotiate these with an owner.

Confidence is key for people to feel change is possible. When smaller changes are successful it can promote an owner's confidence to try bigger, more difficult changes. Therefore, there are advantages to supporting owners to look at smaller, less significant changes, should they choose to do this first. Sometimes, people need to start to work on one change which allows them to realise that the focus actually really needs to be a different or bigger change.

At the other end of the spectrum, some people overestimate their abilities to make changes or underestimate how much work and effort will be required. They may come up with grand schemes for making significant changes, which might not be possible at first. This can lead to a swift discovery that the changes are difficult, do not work or take too much time and energy, causing them to give up all together. For these cases, some techniques for the later stages of the Stages of Change Model, outlined in Chapter 10 (10.5, 10.6), will help them to slow up, consider what might and might not work, and how plans could be adapted to smaller, more manageable chunks (10.6).

6.12   Specific Agenda for a Consultation or a Visit

It is useful to quickly re-establish the agreed overall agenda with the owner at the start of each consultation, visit, or meeting with them. This helps keep both the worker and the owner on track and stay focused. This could be done by saying something such as,

> 'We agreed to look at your dog's weight and how to reduce it. Last time we spoke we agreed that today we would look at his diet. Is that still what we need to focus on or is there something else we need to discuss?'.

This example allows the confirmation of the discussion's agenda, reminding both worker and owner what has been agreed and what the focus will be on a particular day. It also enables the owner to agree to work on the dog's weight and diet or to bring something else in to the discussion. The worker will need to be skilful, still keep to the work in hand and not be distracted or deflected off to other areas. However, this provides an opportunity to allow for something that may have happened since we last saw them and their dog. For example, if the owner has lost their job since the last meeting, that may have an impact on their ability to pay for the recommended special food. On the other hand, it could also mean that they and the dog are taking three long walks a day and thus using the opportunity of having more time to get them both fitter and healthier! This illustrates how checking the agenda, and if necessary changing it, can be very helpful and may even save time in the long run.

6.13   Agenda Mapping

Miller and Rollnick (2013) give a visual way of working with people to identify possible agendas to work on. This agenda mapping can help to pull out and agree specific areas to focus on rather than broad issues such as the health and well-being of the animal. An example of this can be seen in Box 6.2 below. All the circles can be left blank (Box 6.2) to be completed with the owner or, depending on our organisation, role, or purpose of the intervention, some areas can be filled in as suggestions or prompts.

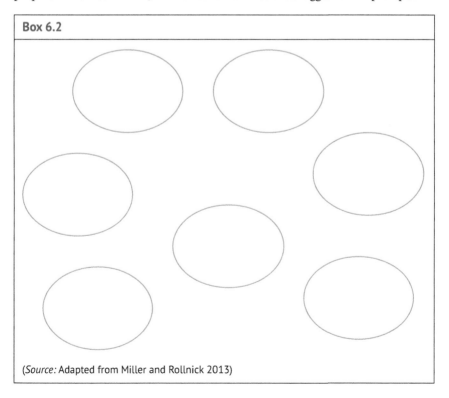

Box 6.2

(*Source:* Adapted from Miller and Rollnick 2013)

An example below might be a semi-prefilled agenda map to start with someone who has a new companion animal such as a puppy or a kitten (Box 6.3).

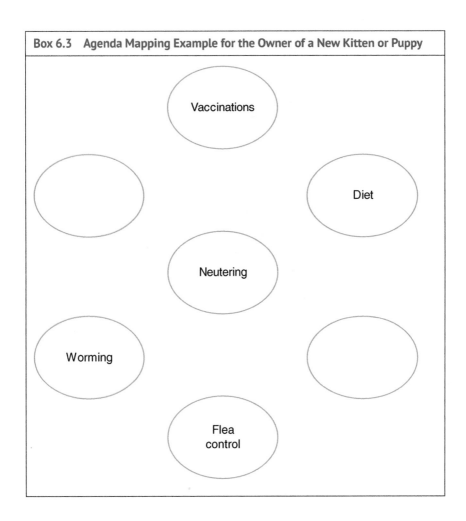

Box 6.3 Agenda Mapping Example for the Owner of a New Kitten or Puppy

Vaccinations

Diet

Neutering

Worming

Flea control

These visual methods of identifying areas to work on and what to start with can be very helpful to many people. Issues being collaboratively mapped and drawn out supports engagement with an owner and underpins the idea of personal choice and responsibility (4.10.4) that is key to the MI approach.

For anyone, thinking about changing behaviours can be overwhelming and it is often difficult to know where to start. A particular behaviour is often linked and inter-woven with other behaviours and it can be difficult to separate them out. I often think about a behaviour as being a cog, with other cogs around it. Often, we need to make changes to one or two of those interlinking cogs to allow us to make a behaviour change. Chunking issues down, by using a tool such an agenda map, can be useful.

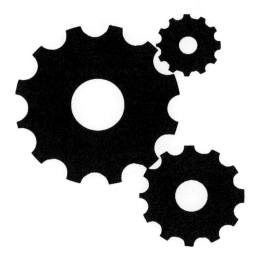

Box 6.4   Exercise

If you would like to try this out for yourself, think about your own behaviours, perhaps a health behaviour (we all usually have a few!). You might think about exercise, weight, diet, sleep, alcohol, or even flossing your teeth. If you were to work on just one behaviour, think about which would you choose and why?

Then consider how your chosen behaviour sits with other things, issues, behaviours: how it fits with the other 'cogs' in your life. For example, weight may be interlinked with exercise, diet, alcohol, and other behaviours. What do you make of what you have thought about?

Agenda maps can seem a bit simplistic, but it is worth thinking about using them. Visual representations of issues can be very helpful for many people. Some owners may have less ability than other people with planning and organising. Agenda mapping may be a way for helping these people to visualise what the issues are. It can be especially useful with people who may have some cognitive problems such as learning disabilities or illnesses such as dementia.

Over 16% of the UK adult population has very poor literacy skills (Literacy Trust), therefore visual representations can be helpful for them. Many people are ashamed of their difficulties with reading and writing and are therefore unlikely to share their problems with professionals. Visual agenda mapping also takes the focus away from the face-to-face nature of the interaction and onto something collaboratively shared by worker and owner. This can reduce pressure and change the dynamic with people who are nervous. It can allow them to take ownership of the discussions. Simple visual tools such as agenda maps can support the conversation to be a more guiding style (5.12.3) of communication rather than the worker directing (5.12.1).

6.14   Agendas – How They Help

Talking about and setting an agenda for a discussion or identifying one for our involvement helps to support animal owners and others to make behaviour changes. As already outlined, agendas can assist with collaborative working, to identify and clarify expectations, and to help minimise misunderstandings, difficulties, and discord (3.8, 4.6) in the conversations and relationship between worker and owner.

Box 6.5   Exercise – Follow, Direct and Guiding in Meetings

*Think about some meetings you may have attended (we have all been to a few!). Imagine a meeting in which there is a clear agenda from the start, and a good chair who carefully steers the meeting to keep to the agenda. The chair may allow a few asides, address some issues brought up by others, especially if urgent, perhaps have some humour and shared jokes, but the agenda is maintained and respected. The chair is interested in people's views and opinions and facilitates these being heard simply and helpfully. These meetings tend to end amicably, time is used wisely, and cake may even be included. The chair's style here could be seen as **guiding** (5.12.3).*

*Now think about the meeting which lacks clarity and form. You, and probably everyone else, are unclear about the exact items to be covered and the reason for the meeting. These types of meetings are often muddled, frustrating, and can involve bad temper with all sorts of issues being aired and few, if any, conclusions or actions agreed upon. They can take more time, and some people may arrive late and leave early, adding to the chaos. If there is cake, it gets eaten by a few people who leave the crumbs behind when they go early. Here the chair may only be using **following** (5.12.2) as a communication style.*

---

*A third type of meeting might be the one in which the agenda is owned by the chair who keeps rigidly to it and allows no deviation from what they believe needs to be covered and the outcomes required. These meetings may not take much time (thankfully), but most of us come out thinking that the information could have been communicated in an email. We may also be less willing to engage in what is required. It is extremely unlikely that there was any cake. **Directing** (5.12.1) is likely to describe this chair's approach.*

What are your experiences of different styles of meetings? Can you identify those that were most useful and used time wisely? Probably such meetings had an agenda that was central, agreed, and although some deviation was allowed, it was respectfully kept on task with everyone feeling engaged. Probably a skilful chair could be seen to be using a guiding communication style for the majority of the meeting, along with occasional directing when required, to get everyone to focus on the matter in hand, not just on the cake. Where directing is mostly or only used, it isn't a meeting, it's an information delivering event.

6.15 Agendas and the Stages of Change

The stages of change (Chapter 3) can give pointers to how workers might identify and work with agendas with owners. In *precontemplation*, it may take a bit of time to listen and guide owners to identify what might be an issue, what could need changing. They probably don't see it as urgent or needing too much attention right now. They may not have the intent to make any changes to their behaviour in the next few months or so.

In the *contemplation* stage, the individual will be experiencing ambivalence (3.4, 4.8). Something probably needs to change but how and when might it change and what will be the cost of changing? Approaching and setting an agenda or focus of the discussion will be different for an owner in the contemplation stage. An owner probably knows some changes are needed but their situation may be complex or muddled, with multiple difficulties or issues to overcome. Here, using agenda mapping and guiding owners to consider the different elements of their animal's health or welfare is time well spent. In fact, in some cases, this may be all that is really needed to be done. Many people, once they have unravelled the tangled ball of string of their difficulties, move swiftly on to the next stages of change; knowing what they need to do. They can shift into *preparation* and goal setting and on to *action*.

In *preparation* stage, the agenda is likely to be very clear and there can now be a move to goal setting (see Chapter 10) around that agenda. Similarly, in *action* and *maintenance,* the agenda is usually clear but may need to be double checked, reaffirmed and possibly tweaked.

Remember, someone may be in one stage of change for one behaviour, but in another stage for a different one. When these different behaviours are linked, or one is required for the other to be successfully changed, agendas may take a bit of work. If we rush and assume the agenda without clarifying this with the owner, problems occur. This can happen when the worker overestimates which stage of change the owner is in at that moment. Workers can similarly underestimate, mistakenly believing that the owner is in an earlier stage of change, causing owners to become frustrated as they want to move forward and thus creating the risk of discord being generated (3.8, 4.6).

Collaboratively agreed agendas allow all parties to keep to the purpose of our professional relationship with the owner. It gives the worker the ability, and permission, to gently guide the owner back to the agreed topic and to focus on the identified issues. A little bit of time spent identifying and confirming an agreed agenda can save a great deal of time and frustration for the rest of the consultation or discussion, as well as future ones. It can help us engage with people and keep a collaborative working relationship (4.10.1), even when difficult conversations are needed. A focus and agenda can support the worker to be neutral (4.10.4) and to avoid slipping into those traditional methods of working with behaviour change.

Agendas help with time keeping and ensure that the time spent with owners is productive. Very often workers in both human health care and in animal health and welfare don't have much time, so agendas really help in their work. Supporting people to consider behaviour changes and the use of MI is more than just being nice (4.2). Yes, we may use our social skills to engage, but keeping these to a minimum allows us to get on with the agreed focus: the agenda.

Box 6.6   Thinking About Agendas

I sometimes think about how working with agendas with humans is rather like how we might set the scene for a walk with our dog or a ride with a horse. It is exciting and the dog or horse, and possibly us, are keen to be off with the possibilities ahead and we risk setting out and going in all directions.

If we are sensible, we will keep the dog on a shorter lead at first, the horse on a tight rein as we start out away from home. Then, as we all settle into the walk or the ride, we can relax a little and loosen the lead or the rein.

Having a conscious and tighter rein or lead allows us to reel things back in quickly and easily should they run away with us. So it is with agendas: they allow workers to bring the conversation back to the matter in hand easily, allowing some digression in case it is useful to the task, but enabling unnecessary and peripheral conversations to be shut down.

Having a clear focus in a conversation, whether in person or by phone, can aid workers to draw back an overtalkative owner or welfare reporter to the required agenda or steer one who moves away from the subject with irrelevant peripheral information. This will be a fine judgement sometimes, as we do need to understand people's perspectives, their experience, frame of reference (Chapter 1) and the backstory to the situation. However, an owner or reporter may have problems focusing, for reasons such as cognitive problems, poor social skills, or perhaps loneliness. An agenda, a focus, allows the worker to kindly but firmly steer the person back to the agreed subject or issue.

A common comment by those coming new to MI is that exploring and agreeing an agenda will take too much time. Repeatedly, the research evidence, and anecdotally from those I have trained, demonstrates that MI makes interventions with individuals quicker, with better outcomes and with less need to keep revisiting cases or issues. Some of the equine welfare officers trained in MI identified that time spent early on by understanding, listening, exploring, and identifying agendas, when done well, allowed the whole process to be speedier overall.

Having agreed focus to the work and conversations with an owner allows the use of the MI techniques we will cover in coming chapters. These techniques do not work well when the interaction lacks focus, is vague or ambiguous.

Agendas also allow us, as workers, to monitor our work and to reflect on our practice (5.10) and supports both workers and owners to be clear about what has been achieved. Therefore, I suggest agendas are central, almost like the hub, of the work that we will do. It is worth coming back to this chapter as you move through the coming chapters and develop more MI techniques.

Box 6.7 Clinical Example

The impact of not identifying and confirming an agenda with an owner is illustrated by the following experience that a welfare colleague gave.

A person that the worker had been supporting had come to the conclusion that the time was very imminent for their old horse to be euthanised.

The owner called their veterinary practice to arrange a visit and the welfare worker could hear the conversation. The owner spoke to the young vet who would come out. The owner told the vet that they wanted a visit to reassess the horse but also that it was very possible that they would need to make the decision to euthanise at that same visit. The owner very clearly laid their agenda out – reassessment and very possibly euthanasia in that visit.

The vet's response was that they were sure that things could be improved, and they would bring some medication out to help with pain relief. The welfare worker's heart sank as they listened. The vet did not hear or try to clarify the owner's agenda. They were not working in a neutral way; rather, they were working to their own agenda, however well meaning. The owner had clearly given their agenda and the vet had not picked this up or addressed it. This was not the best way forward for all involved in this case, including the horse.

6.16 Conclusion

This chapter has outlined the importance of a shared understanding between the worker and the owner for the focus, the agenda, of a conversation. Time spent working on identifying and clarifying agendas makes the work swifter. The specific tools from MI, and from other interventions, work much better if we are clear and agreed about the agenda. Life events and circumstances may mean that agendas for our owners shift and change over time or between consultations or visits. Be ready to check and re-establish the agenda.

Behaviour changes are usually linked to other behaviours. Spend time exploring how the cogs interact to help both you and the owner understand this. You and the owner may agree on an agenda, but then at the next appointment they have realised that they actually need to work on something else first. This is common and often beneficial, so be prepared to guide and work with different issues and changes in direction.

In the next chapters, we will look at more specific techniques, mostly from MI, that can help frame conversations with owners and others. To use these methods to their best advantage, the ideas in this current chapter and the previous ones, especially active listening (Chapter 5), will be needed to underpin what we do. It may be worth coming back to some of the ideas in these first chapters periodically as you consider the methods outlined in the following chapters.

References

Literacy Trust https://literacytrust.org.uk/information/what-is-literacy.

Miller, W.R. and Rollnick, S. (2013). *Motivational Interviewing: Helping People Change,* 3rd ed. New York: Guilford Press.

Miller, W.R. and Rollnick, S. (2023). *Motivational Interviewing: Helping People Change and Grow,* 4th ed. New York: Guilford Press.

7

Three Structures to Understand Behaviours and What Change Might Mean

7.1 Introduction

The previous chapter explored how an agreed focus or agenda is key to supporting people to make behaviour change, especially when using MI. This chapter will look at three specific techniques that can frame and guide conversations with owners and others and help us, and them, develop understanding about their behaviours. These techniques are, firstly, the use of a timeline to look back at how the owner arrived in this situation and secondly, a typical day to explore how behaviours currently fit into their life. Lastly, scaling questions help explore how important (or not) it is for the person to make the change and then what level of confidence they have to make that change.

7.2 Structuring Conversations to Aid Understanding

As covered in the previous chapter, identifying an agenda is different and separate from setting goals (6.6). An agenda brings a focus to our conversation whereas a goal is an outcome. Goals are absolutely appropriate when an owner is in the preparation (3.5) or action (3.6) stages of change. However, when someone is in precontemplation (3.3) or contemplation (3.2), goals are unlikely to be helpful and can be unconstructive.

Supporting people who need to make behaviour changes requires workers to be attentive, and to move with the individual as they contemplate their situation, difficulties, and possibilities. The worker needs to be dancing with an owner rather than wrestling (4.10.1), being reflexive in style (5.10) and able to adapt to the individual moment to moment. However, there is also the need to keep the owner on

Practical Human Behaviour Change for the Health and Welfare of Animals,
First Edition. Bronwen Williams.
© 2024 John Wiley & Sons Ltd. Published 2024 by John Wiley & Sons Ltd.
Companion website: www.wiley.com/go/williams/human

track, supporting them to focus, and to have an agreed agenda about what exactly it is we are considering with them.

This focus, or agenda, is key for the techniques that can help people to explore the behaviours they may need to make. The techniques covered in this chapter and the ones that follow, help the worker to guide (5.12.3) the individual and provide direction for the conversations. This will be helpful not only to the owner but also to the worker. These structures, used flexibly according to the owner's needs, give confidence to workers, helping them to avoid the traditional approaches (outlined in Chapter 2 and that don't really work) or the traps (4.7) which are easy for all of us to fall into.

Box 7.1   Sustain talk and evoking change talk

Sustain talk is the reasons given by a person for not changing, why change would be difficult, why they can't change yet, and why they don't have the intent to change right now.

Change talk is what we hear when people consider a change, no matter how tenuously.

Evoking change talk is where the worker supports the owner to draw out, for themselves, the reasons for possible change. This might be likened to using a poultice to draw out hidden matter that is preventing healing.

The techniques or structures in this chapter all help to evoke change talk from the owner as well as allowing workers to hear and acknowledge sustain talk.

MI techniques, or structures to conversations, allow the owner to explore their ambivalence (3.4), to voice their sustain talk (4.9) and for change talk to be evoked (4.10.1) (Miller and Rollnick 2023). See Box 7.1 above for a brief reminder of these.

The techniques and ideas described in this chapter, and the ones that follow, do not need to be undertaken in a linear way. Rather, they are helpful methods that can be selected in the moment as we see fit while working with an individual. Some of these work well when written down or drawn out at the time with the owner. Workers can also simply hold them in mind to give a mental aid, a structure or framework to conversations.

Using the structures that follow takes a bit of practice. Those to whom we teach MI can feel a bit clumsy and self-conscious when first using them but despite this they still have good outcomes. Often our clients or owners don't realise we are using new techniques. They are too busy considering their position, thoughts and feelings about change. Working with these structures does take a certain amount of reflexivity from the worker and reflection-in-action (5.10). Like most things in life, this all gets easier with practice.

Box 7.2   Using Templates or Drawing Out / Writing Down

In this chapter, three techniques or structures to conversations are explained: timelines, typical day, and exploring importance and confidence scales. It is suggested that some of these are written down or drawn out with the owner. Usually, it is easier if we, as workers, do the writing rather than the owner.

Some of the structures discussed have templates which can be found in Chapter 14. Some workers print and take these into consultations or on visits as blank forms that they can pull out and use if necessary. This works well if you are yet to be completely familiar with them all.

If the owner wants to complete the forms or scales themselves then let them. However, when the worker records, it affords the owner space and time to consider, reflect, and form their thoughts without having to also think about writing information down at the same time. Some people have problems with literacy, and being asked to write something down may fill them with dread, fear or embarrassment and they can disengage. For someone with dyslexia, they too may struggle and consequently concentrate more on feelings of stress than the task at hand. There are, however, some people who think best by writing, drawing, or doodling, so they may need to be the person who writes, alongside their thinking and talking. Workers should still offer or ask if the owner would prefer them to jot notes down. This keeps it collaborative (4.10.1).

The templates are useful, but they are not essential for the use of these techniques. A plain piece of paper will suffice so long as you can remember the structure. I tend to make sure I have a notebook of some sort with me when working with people. Preferably, one that can have pages removed and given to the owner at the end of the conversation as I generally don't keep what has been written down. I give it to the owner; after all, it is their work. It can also serve to remind them of what has been discussed. If you want or need a copy to remind you, ask permission and photocopy it or take a picture with your phone.

When writing down or drawing out some of the following techniques, aim to do so physically alongside the client or owner, allowing them to clearly see what you are doing. Again, this helps with collaborative working (4.10.1) and supports a guiding (5.12.3) style of communication.

Write down what the owner says, use their words, or summarise them and ask if you have got it correct. Avoid using your own interpretation and professional language. For example, if an owner talks about their previous dogs, their illnesses and that they all had 'weight issues', the worker should record the owner's language. If the worker interprets and writes down 'obesity', it may easily have a significant impact on the owner and on how they feel about continuing the discussion.

7.3 Timeline

The first structure we might chose is a timeline. Timelines can be used for an initial exploration of the agreed agenda, but can also be used at other times or once done, returned to when needed. Timelines are not a method from MI; rather, it is a finetuned form of an activity that we all will be familiar with, that of taking a history. However, a timeline is different from the usual history-taking in two fundamental and essential ways.

First, it is the client or owner who creates the timeline, their version of the history, rather than the usual approach in which when histories are taken, we or other professionals lead and direct it.

Second, the timeline is focused on the current agenda as identified and agreed with the client or owner (Chapter 6). This means that, rather than a broad professional history-taking, a timeline is specifically focused and narrowed on the issue of concern or the behaviour change that is being explored.

Box 7.3   Timelines Are Already Part of Our Work

Many of us in both human and animal health care use timelines for many things, including incident investigation when something has gone wrong. When we take any type of history from an owner or client, we use some sort of timeline. For example, we often ask when did this start, when did you first notice it, what happened then? So, this technique is familiar for us to use when trying to get information, sift and sort that material to make sense of it, and then find a diagnosis or an answer.

When history-taking, we do just that: we take or extract information from the other person. We are in control of the conversation and are in the role of an expert. When professionals lead a timeline discussion, or extract a history, the owner will often report only what they think we need or want to hear, and so, important details can be left out. With the spirit of the approach of MI, the use of the timeline shifts away from workers being investigators aiming to find the answers. Rather, the worker supports and guides the owner to do the investigating, to see if <u>they</u> can come up with the answers.

Those from animal welfare work using MI for behaviour change have frequently reported that the use of the timeline has been one of the most impactful strategies for the owners they work with. Use of the timeline alone can bring significant insights, often leading owners to have increased motivation to change. The timeline can prompt sustain talk (4.9) and evoke change talk (4.10.2) thus opening up dialogue and generating useful information. Timelines support the worker to then guide the individual and to use some of the other techniques outlined in this chapter and the following ones.

7.4   Using a Timeline with an Owner or Client

Undertaking a timeline should, as always, be conversational in manner, with the worker curious, neutral (4.10.4) and ensuring that a clear focus or agenda (Chapter 6) has been established with the owner. If a collaborative agenda (6.9) is not in place, the timeline is unlikely to work well. Rather, the conversation could dissolve into a general chat, which can be bewildering for the owner and makes it difficult for the worker to bring focus back and to use guiding (5.12.3) as a communication style.

A timeline doesn't need to be done all in one go: it can be returned to at a later date and added to. A completed timeline may also be returned to later to review and support the individual's ideas and thinking. On occasions, some owners add to their timelines outside appointments with workers and then bring these back to support further discussions.

Written down or drawn out timelines can allow people to see their experiences in black and white in front of them. Below is an example of a timeline given by a first-time owner with an overweight dog.

As you can see, the worker has written down what the owner has told them; this would have been done physically alongside the owner as they were speaking. Our role as worker is not to point out what the owner 'did wrong' or 'got right' but rather to use active listening to support the owner to explore, out loud, their circumstances and how they got to this point.

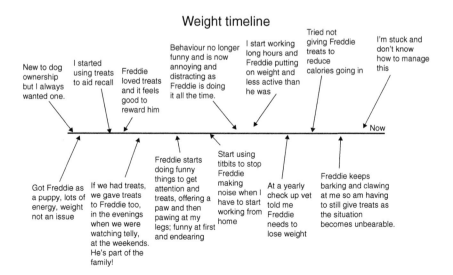

Weight timeline

Below is a more complex timeline that might be typical for someone who has been struggling with their animals, equines in this case, and has slid into a situation that would meet the criteria for animal hoarding, specifically 'overwhelmed caregiver hoarding' (Williams 2014).

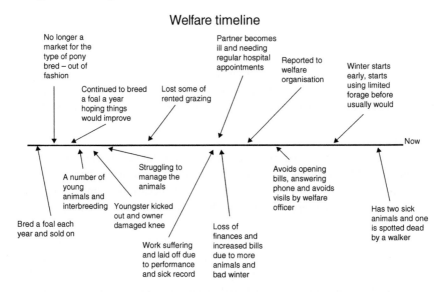

The owner can start to see things more clearly which can really support them to consider and decide what changes might be made. Timelines can also help the workers, as well as owners, understand how the current situation came about. This can help us have more empathy (5.15) with owners, even in difficult welfare cases.

Box 7.4   When Using a Timeline – Things to Avoid

Avoid pointing what the owner did wrong.
Avoid pointing out when things did go right.
Avoid making connections (rather, through active listening, encourage the owner to make any connections and invite them to join the dots).
Avoid drawing conclusions (rather, guide the owner to do this themself as then it is much more powerful and helpful).

Each timeline will be different. In some, there may be possibilities for the owner to identify what has worked for them in the past and so build their confidence for behaviour changes that might now need to be made.

Owners may be able to identify what has tripped them up in previous behaviour change attempts, as well as the issues or events that led to the current situation. This type of information can be returned to when the owner moves into preparation for change and needs ideas about how to plan do so. Details uncovered in timelines can be invaluable for planning change and so help owners to avoid or manage potential pitfalls (10.12).

A timeline can be a little like a dot-to-dot picture. We are asking the individual to identify the dots themselves, and then we are inviting and guiding them to join the dots to see the whole picture. It is common for many of us, when experiencing a difficult situation, worry or issue, to think about it frequently but keep it to ourselves. However, when given support to speak about it or write it down in some way, we can often see the whole picture, perhaps for the first time, and so gain more understanding or a different perspective. In some cases, there may also be the flexibility to do more than one timeline, perhaps where there are several behaviour changes required over time.

With the example of the person who slid into hoarding in timeline 2 above, no dates were given. Some people may give years or dates or other things that may frame their timeline. It doesn't really matter. What does matter is that you record what is said in the owner's words, to structure their memory and exploration of the issue. One person I worked with in my human health role had for many years skippered boats. He used the names of different boats to structure his memory and timeline for a particular issue we were exploring.

Box 7.5 Exercise – Try It for Yourself – Join the Dots

Quickly draw out a timeline with your work history on it. Instead of writing it down as is usual for a job application or a CV, make notes using the timeline of anything that was pertinent to you at the time. Perhaps add what made you change roles, how this came about. What else was significant in your life at those points on your timeline? Add anything in that is relevant to you and your experience.

Now, take a few minutes to look at what you have drawn out. Add anything else that you think of. Do you notice any themes or highlights? Perhaps things you hadn't quite noticed before or couldn't put your finger on? Any dots to be joined?

Note, this exercise is for a timeline without someone else to support or guide you through it. Timelines are designed to be facilitated by a supportive listener. So, if you can find someone to do this for you, who can be neutral and not fall into traditional methods, ask them to help you and see what a difference that support can make.

7.5 Timelines in Use – Experiences from Welfare Workers

Animal welfare colleagues I have trained often report back that the timeline has made some of the biggest impact on their work. When timelines have been used to support owners and others to change behaviours for the welfare of their animals, workers found that it helped them structure their conversations and supported the underpinning spirit of the MI approach. However, when the timeline was used as a standalone task and without the spirit of MI or good active listening (5.13), curiosity, and neutrality (4.10.4), the outcomes were poorer.

Box 7.6   When Using a Timeline – Do...
Ensure you have a clear focus (agenda). Use the agenda to keep you, the owner and the timeline to what has been agreed. Invite the owner to consider their experience. Ask open questions such as: 'What do you make of this now?' 'What has tripped you up / got in the way in the past?' 'Where have you been successful in making change in the past?' 'When you consider your past experiences, what do you think might help you in the future?' 'Is there anything else you want to add?'

One of these colleagues who used the timeline successfully, described how they undertook it in a conversation while walking across a field with an owner. It helped both the worker and owner understand the situation. They reported that by using a timeline, they found out a great deal in 20 minutes, much of which wouldn't have come to light without it. Other animal workers say that not only does the timeline allow the owner to explore what has happened to create the current situation, but very often it allows the owner themselves to start to identify the issues. This is what MI is about: the individual identifying concerns for themselves, and talking themselves into any changes that might be made.

Box 7.7   Exercise – Try It for Yourself
You could think about a behaviour of your own that you might explore: a health behaviour, perhaps, such as exercise or alcohol or smoking, if you have ever smoked. It can be a behaviour you currently do, one you have done in the past, or one that you have started and stopped a number of times. Remember to have a focus, or an agenda, a specific behaviour, and draw out a timeline for yourself.

See what you notice.

What do you make of it?

Are there any dots you can join?

Are there any patterns that you can see?

This may not work so well as having someone talk you through it, but it may be interesting to try.

Box 7.8   Exercise – Practice Before You Use a Timeline with a Client or Owner

Perhaps you might practice a timeline with someone else before using it within your work or professional role.

You could ask a friend or family member to help you practice and to work through a timeline of theirs.

Often people are very happy to talk about a health behaviour that they would like to explore or even change.

If there are no health behaviour changes that they can come up with, perhaps ask them to do with you a timeline of their educational experiences or their career and job roles.

Another agenda for timelines that I often use in training is to ask people if they might do a timeline of the animals they have had in their life (this one can be rather emotional so be prepared for that, but it is also a lovely one).

7.6   Typical Day

Another way to structure conversations around behaviour change is to use a typical day. It is a useful technique, and although it won't necessarily fit with every piece of work or every owner, it can be used, where appropriate, in earlier conversations about change. However, you can always return to it, or use it for the first time, later on in the process should you feel that it might be valuable.

Again, the agenda needs to be clear before you use the typical day. If the agenda is broad and non-specific, the typical day, as with the other methods that give structure, will be less successful, and it will be much easier to get lost and fall into the traps (4.7).

The typical day needs to be done in a conversational manner, but not as a sociable chat. Clarify the agenda and then use a *guiding* (5.12.3) style to assist the person to keep on task, keeping to the agreed agenda. Allow some digression, which may give useful information, but know when to shut down unproductive peripheral chat.

7.7 How to Use a Typical Day

When there is a clear agenda about the focus of the conversation, you can ask the owner or the client to talk you through their typical day and where the behaviour fits into it.

Prompt for as much detail as possible and allow them to describe and explore anything around the particular behaviour.

Box 7.9   Typical Day – Start Example

WORKER: 'Could you talk me through your typical day and when feeding Sandy happens in it?'

OWNER: 'Well, Sandy will be wanting his breakfast as soon as I wake up. Sometimes, he wakes me up to tell me it's breakfast time!'

WORKER: 'Around what time would that be?'

OWNER: 'For me, around 6.30 in the morning is usual, but Sandy has been waking me up from before 6 sometimes. It is a real pain!'

WORKER: 'Sometimes, Sandy wakes you up before you are ready!' (reflecting), 'What happens next...?'

For a Welfare Case – some questions to start the typical day
Could you tell me about a typical day for you and how looking after your animals fits into that?
When do you start?
What happens?
What next?

Sometimes, just from talking through their typical day, an owner realises that the agenda and their attention and focus needs to be on a different area or issue than originally thought. Those who are in precontemplation (3.3) may start to realise that there <u>are</u> issues of concern or some which need consideration. This may be quite a shock for an owner, especially as they are saying this out loud, not only to themselves, but also to another person. Now, we can see why all those skills of active listening (5.2), of being neutral (4.10.4) and flexible and focusing on the process rather than the outcome (not goal setting) (4.10.1) can be so important here.

Ask the person to start describing what happens in their day and occurs before the issue you are discussing. If the issue you are focusing on occurs later in the day, then start a while before that. Although you probably won't need to know absolutely everything that happens from very early on in their day, some information before the behaviour happens will be useful, but use your judgement. The focus of an agreed agenda will help keep both the owner and the worker on track with information relevant to the behaviour under discussion.

Use prompts and all your active listening skills, especially reflecting (simple and complex 5.16), mini summaries (5.17), and non-verbal prompts (5.5) to encourage the owner to explore. Asking about their typical day allows you to understand the context of the issues and behaviours for the individual, other behaviours that may interact or inter-relate, and also other people who may have an influence on what does, or doesn't, happen.

If, for example, the agreed agenda is around diet and feeding an animal, you will get information about how this fits into the person's life. You may get some hints about their frame of reference (Chapter 1). Perhaps you start to hear the idea that they hate to see an animal hungry and so feed them treats and titbits. Or maybe a belief that food should not be wasted so anything that family members leave at a meal is given to the dog. You never know until you ask and then listen.

Sometimes, it can be worth exploring a typical *week*, depending on how the issue lends itself to being examined.

Box 7.10   Prepare to Be Surprised

Kelly, one of my human health co-training colleagues used typical day routinely with prisoners when she was working as a nurse in a prison health care setting. It would have been easy to assume that all prisoners' typical days would be the same due to the rigid structure within these institutions. That was not the case, and each prisoner had a different view and experience of their days in incarceration and could articulate very different meanings. She would often then ask them to compare and contrast: a typical day in prison and then what their typical day had been prior to starting their sentence. We can now start to see the wealth of information that can be elicited from this technique when used as a structure but used creatively and underpinned by supportive active listening, curiosity, and exploration.

Box 7.11   Typical Day – Welfare Example

One animal welfare colleague used the typical day and found out that a horse owner was making regular daily visits to her horses. However, they also discovered that when the owner felt overwhelmed and unable to cope with the escalating welfare issues, she just glanced at the horses as she drove past the field and didn't stop. The welfare worker may well not have found this out without asking about the owner's typical day.

Remember, the typical day can be used flexibly to meet the focus of the conversation and the needs of the owner. Issues may only be present at distinct times, such as specific seasons or weather, or when something particular impacts upon the individual or their circumstances.

Another way of using typical day is to explore when problems occur at particular times, perhaps at a weekend, or when the person does or doesn't have company for example. Again, like the example above of my colleague working in the prison, you could ask about a typical day when things tend to go right as well as a typical day when things are problematic or impact upon animal welfare. It could perhaps be a typical day in the winter and one in summer. Those of us with larger animals know that typical days in different seasons can be very different!

When you first start using a typical day, it is often easier to initially use it with behaviours that need to be taken out rather than added in. For example, a typical day around not giving a companion animal food outside of mealtimes may be easier to try than, say, increasing the exercise your client gives an animal, but this is a rough rule. With practice and experimentation, you will find you can use typical day in all sorts of ways and with all types of behaviours: you can adapt and be creative for different people and their issues.

7.8 Tips to Aid Typical Day

Remember
- Try and guide the person to focus on the agreed agenda.
- But do allow them to wander a little; don't keep them too tightly tied to the identified issue as other information can be illuminating to both you and them.
- Ask for details.
- Don't assume. Everyone does things differently, so ask the obvious.
- Be curious, be neutral, be kind.
- Be creative with a typical day, to suit what the owner is telling you and what their issue is.
- Guide the conversation by slowing down if particular elements may be worth exploring more, and speeding up the discussion (Rollnick 2006) if the person is stuck in the minutia of everyday life and giving details that don't add to or relate to the overall picture.

Box 7.12   Give Prompts, Including Open Questions, Alongside Reflections

You can say things like the following.
How does that fit into your typical day?
What happens then?
How does that impact your day?
How does that work for you?
What do you make of that?

Box 7.13   Example of Typical Day in Use

An example of how a typical day unexpectedly gave me surprising but useful information was when I was covering visits for an NHS human mental health colleague who was on leave. I had to deliver medication and administer an injection to someone I had not met before but who was well known to the service and to the excellent nurse who usually saw her. To help build a rapport and engagement, I asked the patient about her life and how she occupied herself and found myself in a typical day conversation. For some reason, the patient's mention of coffee stood out, and as she told me about her day, I realised that it was punctuated by very frequent mugs of coffee. In the end, I asked, out of curiosity, how many coffees she would drink during the typical day. The answer was around 40. This was when I realised that her complaints of anxiety and sleeplessness, although she had a primary diagnosis of psychosis, may have a very obvious cause. We went on to discuss how coffee might be affecting her and what she thought she might change.

Box 7.14   Exercise – Practice Typical Day on Someone Easier at First (learn with a small car before you move on to a Ferrari)

You might like to try out a typical day with someone such as a friend or a colleague before you use the technique with a client or owner.

Remember to be upfront and honest about what you are doing and what it is that you are asking them to do.

Ask if they would be prepared to help you practice, and then identify an agreed agenda with them, the behaviour that they are happy to discuss: most people will be delighted to talk to you about their own health and what issues they have with it.

Remember that you may need to spend time helping the person identify and clarify exactly what the issues might be and what the agenda is. They might identify multiple issues and you will need to ask which in particular they would like to focus on first.

Remember to integrate all those active listening skills into the conversation about a typical day: reflecting (simple and complex 5.16) and summarising (5.17), reducing questions to a minimum, and when you do ask questions, try to use open rather than closed questions (5.14). Think about being neutral (4.10.4), about guiding (5.12.3) and not coming up with suggestions or ideas but rather going with the process and not chasing an outcome (4.10.1).

When you have finished the typical day practice, ask your friend or colleague for feedback. Find out about their experience and what you did that was helpful and what you might have done differently.

Reflect yourself (reflection-on-action 5.10) about what worked and you would use again and what you might do differently next time to support use of a typical day, whether that be in your work with an owner or in another practice with a friend or colleague about their own personal health behaviours.

7.9   Further Reading

You may like to read some further information that Rollnick has written about using the typical day, which can be found here https://www.nyscha.org/files/2011/handouts/WE-PRE%201%20MI_Typical-Day_Rollnick.pdf

7.10   Exploring Importance and Confidence

Another MI structure or framework to support behaviour change conversations is the use of scaling questions (Miller and Rollnick 2013). With this tool, the individual is invited to explore the behaviour as agreed in the agenda and to consider how important it is for them to change and then how confident they are to make a change. Importance has been described as the 'why of change' whereas confidence is the 'how of change' (Mason 2019). In conversations it is very common to hear people voice why change is, or is not, important and also how confident they are about attempting, or actually making, a change. These are two crucial issues for behaviour change. The scales described here are a great way to help focus on importance and confidence, to bring out more information and to give structure to exploring these in detail.

Box 7.15   Exercise

Before we move onto the structures to explore importance and confidence, think about the following for yourself.

Imagine if you were thinking about making a change in your own life. If you felt it was important to do and you were confident about implementing it – how would that be? What would be likely to happen?

Now, what about if you felt a change was important but you were not confident right now in making it?

What if you felt a change was not important but you were confident you could make it?

And lastly, if you felt it was not important and you had no confidence to make the change?

What do you make of your answers?

Now read on...

A good way of introducing 'importance' and 'confidence' into the conversation is to remind the owner of the agenda to help guide them to focus and to stay on track. Then ask them about their importance, and then confidence, for the change 'right now'. Something like this,

> *'Thinking about your dog's weight, right now, today, how important is it to make changes around this?'*

And then,

> *'Thinking about your dog's weight, right now, today, how confident are you about making changes?'*

Using the immediacy of here and now helps focus and can bring the behaviour change into the spotlight. Owners may then talk about how it might be possible in the future or what is currently different than in the past. This can be significant information and adds to the discussion. When workers ask about 'right now', it allows owners to identify what would need to happen for them to make a change. Using 'right now' gives opportunities to explore and make comparisons around situations, beliefs, and expectations from both the past and the future in addition to where the individual sees themselves in the present moment.

After discussing importance and then the confidence an owner has around a possible change, a third scaling question may be used:

> 'How *ready*, right now, today, are you to make a change... ?'

However, this readiness question may not be useful to ask if you feel it would cause the owner to back off, feel pressure, or it would not be helpful to them at the time. Perhaps, if someone is further along in the stages of change, then it may be appropriate to ask about readiness, but do so carefully and tentatively. I often think of the readiness element as a broad overall discussion and the importance and confidence elements as more specific. More detail about how to use each of these scales can be found below.

Asking about and exploring importance and confidence, and perhaps readiness, can be done at an early stage in the conversation once the agenda has been identified. It can also be returned to if you feel stuck, when you need to regain a structure to the conversation or just at any time it feels right to reuse it. One such time is if you get a sense that someone has moved within the stages of change.

However, the main purpose for these questions is to provide a supportive framework to conversations, to give structure alongside all your active listening skills (5.11), neutrality (4.10.4) and curiosity. Inviting the person to think and talk about the importance for them and then their confidence in making a behaviour change can produce sustain talk (4.9) and also evoke change talk (4.10.2). It can help the owner understand and explore their ambivalence (3.4) about changes that might be made. Remember, the ratio of change talk to sustain talk can indicate where in the stages of change the individual is at that moment. More sustain talk may be heard in the precontemplation (3.3) and in the contemplation (3.4) stages. Less sustain talk and more change talk is heard in the preparation stage and onwards (3.5–3.6).

7.11   Using Scales to Explore Importance, Confidence, and Possibly Readiness

Miller and Rollnick (2013) suggest the use of scales (or what they call rulers) to help frame and structure these conversations.

Importance

← not important   very important →

0	1	2	3	4	5	6	7	8	9	10

Confidence

← not confident   very confident →

0	1	2	3	4	5	6	7	8	9	10

Readiness

← not ready   very ready →

0	1	2	3	4	5	6	7	8	9	10

The scales can either be numbered, usually 0 to 10, or be a little looser, using 'not important' at one end and 'very important' at the other, and for confidence, 'not at all confident' and 'very confident', as shown. Templates of these scales can be printed by the worker to bring out and use with owners when appropriate, or they can be drawn out by the worker during a conversation on some paper that is to hand. They can also simply be used verbally. The worker will need to judge which method to use with an owner. Again, many people value a visual way of working and this can have an impact on them. Working together on a visual scale can also be a very collaborative activity, aiding engagement and the working relationship.

These scales are designed to give structure to conversations and to help owners explore their behaviour and for workers to hear sustain talk, evoke change talk, and to work with ambivalence. As with the previous techniques described in this chapter, these scales need to be undertaken in a conversational manner using active listening (Chapter 5), with neutrality (4.10.4) professional curiosity and empathy (5.15) from the worker.

When you start using these scales, concentrate more on the discussion you have with the person and the information gained rather than the numbers or scores. Often, when we are new to this, we tend to focus on the scores and rush the process. Take your time, be relaxed and curious and remember: process not outcome (4.10.1).

Box 7.16   A Word of Warning

Sometimes, these scales are applied without the other key elements and the spirit of the approach of MI and in ways for which they were never designed; just as rating scales rather than as a structure for a conversation. This can happen when workers or organisations are chasing outcome measures or using these scales, wrongly, to indicate who they should and should not work with. Using the scales in this way is not MI, is unhelpful and can be destructive to engagement with someone who wants or needs to make a behaviour change.

I have seen the scales added to assessment paperwork as a tick box exercise. The person might be asked to rate themselves on the scales without a conversation about what this means to them. This doesn't really get the worker and the owner very far, and it is not in the spirit of MI (4.5). These scales, when used without the underlying spirit of MI, become a blunt assessment tool with little meaning or worth. I have even heard of workers just handing them out to clients and telling them to fill them in. Again, this is not how these scales are designed to be used.

Do make sure you clearly introduce the scales and what they mean. Remind yourself and the owner of the agreed agenda for the discussion. Invite them to explore the possible behaviour change by using some simple scales and explain, if you are using numbers, what '0' means and what '10' means. Use your 'reflection-in-action' (5.10) to monitor any impulses in you to try to lead the owner in any way. Be observant of any indications that the owner is just giving the answers they think you want or would like, rather than what they really think and feel.

7.12   Using the Scaling Questions

Invite the owner to answer some questions about how they feel about or view any possible change. Explain that you are going to ask them about the behaviour that is the agreed agenda, and you will ask them to identify where they might think they are on a scale right now, today.

7.13 Importance (the Why)

We might say,

> *'Right now, today, on a scale of 0 to 10, how important is it to change to this behaviour, 0 being not at all important and 10 being very important'.*

Or, ask them,

> *'If this end is not important, and the other end is very important, where would you place yourself right now, today, on this line?'*

Importance

← not important   very important →

0	1	2	3	4	5	6	7	8	9	10

Remain curious and let them decide; do not try to persuade or cajole for a higher number. When they have given you a score, or a place on the importance scale, ask them to tell you more about where they have placed themselves and why.

Build this into a conversation and guide them to stay on track while allowing exploration of their feelings, beliefs, and thoughts. It is often interesting what will come up here. I have found that when discussing the importance, or not, of behaviour change, people can become quite emotional which can be a surprise for them. Listen and use simple and complex reflections (5.16) to give back to them any sustain talk (4.9) and to allow them to feel heard. Also listen and reflect back any change talk (4.10.2), so hearing and reflecting both sides of their ambivalence (4.8).

In addition to reflecting you may want to add in mini summaries (5.17) to help them capture their thoughts. Use a guiding style (5.12.3) to support all of this.

Often, people will talk about the importance of a change they could make, not to them but for others in their life. This is always worth exploring. You can then expand the conversation about the importance, or not, to the owner of changing the behaviour.

You may find that the conversation for the owner focuses on the importance of the status quo, of staying the same. For example, when an animal is coming to the end of life and the quality of their life is deteriorating, the owner may still need to talk about the importance of having the animal in their life. A simple reflection might be,

WORKER: 'Freddie is a really *important* part of your life.'
OWNER: 'Yes he is, but also, you know this is really hard, because I want the best for him and I don't want his last days to be bad and for him to be suffering.'

Here a double-sided reflection (5.16) might be used such as,

WORKER: 'On the one hand, Freddie is really important to you and you can't imagine how you will be without him, *and* on the other, it is important to you that he has a good quality of life and you don't want that compromised.'

Remember that the owner will need to generate what is important, not the worker. The fundamental premise of MI is, if change is to happen, it is the owner who talks themselves into it. Other people trying to push someone into change will not work, and it may result in increased sustain talk (4.9) and an increased desire to keep the current situation, to maintain the status quo, thus making change less likely.

You can ask questions around the importance scale to help the owner explore further. It is really worth asking what would make this issue more important on the scale. When asking this, it should be in small increments, perhaps one number up on the scale (see box below for examples). Too big an increment and the owner is likely to back off. We can also ask about why the owner didn't place their importance slightly lower down the scale. While this can feel counterintuitive when trying to support the person to move towards change, it can actually often evoke some really interesting and powerful change talk from the individual.

Box 7.17   Exploring Importance – What We Might Ask the Owner

- Tell me about why you placed yourself here on the scale right now?
- How would this become any more important to you / is there anything that would make this more important?
- What would have to be different to move this up the importance scale a little for you? Or what would move you from say, the 6 where you put yourself today, to a 7?
- Why not a lower number? Say a 3 instead of your 6?
- What concerns do you have about changing?
- If it did become more important, what would that be like?
- What do you make of this?

(adapted from Miller and Rollnick 2013)

Simple questions work best with these scales. Remember to stay neutral (4.10.4), curious, flexible and to dance (4.10.1) with the owner as they may well move back and forth within the stages of change, demonstrated by both sustain (4.9) and change (4.10.2) talk.

If someone feels that a change is not at all important for them there may be little reason to expend the energy in making a change. If you do get a very low number from the owner on the importance scale, this can still be useful. Perhaps they don't see the issue as important, but others do, and that can be helpful information. It could be that the agenda or focus of the conversation needs to be changed, and we need to be flexible. It isn't unusual for people to start to explore one area of concern to suddenly realise and say,

> OWNER: '*You know, this really isn't important now I think about it... but what is important is...*'

Here, we might help them to refocus and reset the agenda by saying,

> WORKER: '*Is that something that you would rather talk about right now as that sounds more important to you?*'

7.14 Confidence (the How)

Confidence

← not confident   very confident →

0	1	2	3	4	5	6	7	8	9	10

Next, we can ask the owner how confident they are right now to make the change. This is the confidence to make the specific change in behaviour that is being discussed rather than a general sense of confidence. Ask them what would make them a point or so higher, or more confident. Often, people can rate themselves fairly highly on importance but lower on confidence (think about your answers to the importance and confidence exercise earlier). Confidence fits with the idea of self-efficacy (11.15) or the sense of self-belief that one can do something. Confidence can sometimes be the area that needs the most exploration and work before people can move into making a change. Coming chapters will give ideas on how to help people build confidence in making a change.

Box 7.18   Build Confidence – What We Might Ask the Owner

What would make you more confident about change?

- Why have you placed yourself at that particular point on this scale?
- How could you move up a little, (e.g. say, from 3 where you have put yourself to perhaps 4?)
- Why not a lower number? Say a 3 instead of your 6?
- How can I help you succeed?
- Who else might help you?

(adapted from Miller and Rollnick 2013)

Often, a major reason people haven't made a change or changes is due to a lack of confidence (think back to the exercise above in Box 7.15, where you thought about importance and confidence for you, or perhaps quickly do that exercise now). Owners may have made attempts to change in the past which haven't worked. Human nature is to look at past attempts and say to ourselves, 'There is no point putting myself thorough that again as I failed last time'.

As the worker, it is helpful to keep in mind that this is very usual. As discussed in Chapter 3, the Stages of Change Model tells us that people may need to go through the stages more than once, sometimes several or even many times before a change sticks for them (3.9).

If you get a sense that the owner is focusing on what they see as past failures, the timeline (7.3) may be worth doing for the first time, or revisiting if it was done previously. Timelines allow people to identify what helped and what didn't in past attempts to make a behaviour change.

It can also be useful to listen out for changes that the person has successfully made in the past, even if it is not related to the current behaviour, and discuss those with them. Exploring what worked previously helps people to see change as possible. They can tap into previous skills, knowledge and help they had and so think about what could similarly help them now. This builds self-efficacy (the belief a person has in their ability to change 11.15). Confidence to make a change and self-efficacy are interrelated.

7.15   Readiness

Readiness to Change

← not ready					unsure					ready →
0	1	2	3	4	5	6	7	8	9	10

Once importance (the why) and confidence (the how) have been explored, you might ask about readiness, using a scale, as above. Remind the owner to think about, right now, today, how ready they are to make a change. Beware, however, of encouraging people to score themselves a bit higher or a situation in which the person gives a higher score in an attempt to please you. Ask them similar questions to those asked with importance and confidence.

Box 7.19   Readiness to Change – What We Might Ask the Owner

What would make you more ready to change?

- Why have you placed yourself at that particular point on this scale?
- How could you move up a little, (e.g. say, 3 where you have put yourself to perhaps 4?)

- Why not a lower number? Say a 3 instead of your 6?
- How can I help you succeed?
- Who else might help you?

Asking an owner about readiness could mean that you get ahead of them, from their position at that moment in the stages of change. Consequently they may back off, and it may generate more sustain talk (about why they can't change or need to stay the same) (4.9) than evoking change talk (4.10.2). So, go cautiously with asking about readiness but when the time is right it can be very useful.

Box 7.20   Top Tip

These scales can frame a whole conversation with someone. If you find you are just asking for numbers, are getting little or no detail and the scales are done quickly, then you will need to review how you are using them. These scales are designed to aid exploration, help evoke change talk (4.10.2), increase motivation to change, and aid the understanding of the owner and the worker about the situation.

Box 7.21   An Exercise

You might once again find a friend, colleague or family member to help you practice the use of these scales prior to applying them in your work role.

Ask the person if they would like to discuss a behaviour with you for, say, 15 to 20 minutes. Then work through the scales with them.

Remember, you may need to do a little work first to help them identify or firm up an agenda. If your practice client says, 'I want to be happy!' or 'I want to be healthy!', you will need to encourage them, through a guiding conversation, to identify a clearer focus or agenda (not a goal, although they may mention one) that you can work on together.

Remember to introduce and explain the scales to them and what the numbers or each end of the scales represent.

Use all your best active listening, stay neutral, and curious to help the person to explore the issue using the scales as a structure for the conversation.

Listen out for sustain talk and acknowledge it, listen too for change talk and draw this out using reflections (simple and complex).

The scales really lend themselves to the worker doing mini summaries to feedback change talk and to keep the person on track.

7.16 Conclusion

This chapter has looked at three methods that help to give structure to conversations with owners about change: timeline, typical day and importance, confidence (and readiness) scales. These are useful to use earlier on in the conversations about change, but they can be used at any stage where you feel appropriate. They can also be returned to, again when it feels useful to do so. Timelines and the scales work well when written down, usually by the worker as the owner is talking. However, the structures can also be used to frame and guide our conversations without being documented.

These are not assessment tools to be applied to or used on the owner. Rather, they frame conversations and active listening is essential. All the underlying ideas and principles of MI outlined in earlier chapters need to be applied by the worker. Practice is required for these structures as they often don't come naturally. Although they may look simple, the more they are used, and reflected-on-action (5.10) upon, the better the work with owners will be. This is very much the case with another structure which is covered in the next chapter: exploring ambivalence.

References

Mason, P. (2019) *Health Behaviour Change: A Guide for Practitioners.* 3rd ed. Edinburgh: Elsevier Ltd.

Miller, W.R. and Rollnick, S. (2023) *Motivational Interviewing: Helping People Change and Grow*, 4th ed. New York: Guilford Press.

Miller, W.R. and Rollnick, S. (2013) *Motivational Interviewing: Helping People Change*, 3rd ed. New York: Guilford Press.

Rollnick, S. (2006) Liven up Your Assessment Using a 'Typical Day'. https://www.nyscha.org/files/2011/handouts/WE-PRE%201%20MI_Typical-Day_Rollnick.pdf.

Williams, B. (2014) Animal hoarding – recognition and possible interventions. *In Practice* 36 (4): 199–205.

8

Working with Ambivalence – The Key to Making Change

8.1   Introduction

The previous chapter explored specific techniques that can support and aid conversations. They can give structure and direction to discussions about change for the health, welfare and well-being of people's animals. All the three strategies discussed in the previous chapter – a timeline, a typical day, and scales to explore importance, confidence, and overall readiness for making change – will generate information for both the worker and the owner and highlight ambivalence. By using these you will hear both sustain talk and change talk and will probably experience an owner moving back and forth in the stages of change as they ponder and consider their particular situation, their experiences, beliefs, and values.

Exploring ambivalence is central to MI and the resolution of it is key to behaviour change. This chapter focuses on exploring ambivalence and a framework to support conversations to do this. Exploring ambivalence with an owner can draw out useful information. This chapter will look at some specific issues or areas where exploring ambivalence can be used in animal welfare, health, and care work. It is suggested that you come back to this chapter more than once to reread some of the information as you begin to practice with owners.

The use of the strategies described in the previous chapter (Chapter 7), alongside the MI spirit of approaching conversations, will have built engagement, rapport and hopefully a willingness in the owner to talk and explore. You will remember the importance of evoking change talk and the reasons for change. We aim to use a guiding style to support the individual to pull out, generate their own reasons for change and to talk themselves into the change. It is also important to hear and acknowledge any sustain talk; the reasons why they are in the current situation and what it is about the current behaviour that works for them.

Practical Human Behaviour Change for the Health and Welfare of Animals,
First Edition. Bronwen Williams.
© 2024 John Wiley & Sons Ltd. Published 2024 by John Wiley & Sons Ltd.
Companion website: www.wiley.com/go/williams/human

Exploring and resolving ambivalence is key to making a change for anyone and ambivalence is heard when the person gives the arguments both for, and against, change. There will be reasons to stay the same, to keep the status quo, and these will be voiced through sustain talk. There will also be the other side of the argument within the owner: the reasons for change which are voiced in change talk. Therefore, much of helping people consider a behaviour change is enabling them to explore ambivalence with their reasons for and against change. If possible we will help them strengthen their reasons for change, by hearing and acknowledging their sustain talk and by evoking and expanding their change talk.

8.2   Exploring Ambivalence

The strategy covered in this chapter is one for exploring that ambivalence. It gives the opportunity to look at the behaviour from all angles, consider it in 360 degrees, or in the round. This helps workers move away from those traditional approaches (Chapter 2) of trying to push people to change. Traditional methods have a narrow focus and thus generate neither the richness of detail nor the important, often essential, information that will enable the owner to move towards and make change.

MI gives a framework to explore ambivalence which provides structure to conversations with an owner. It is meant to be used in a conversational manner. It is not designed as formulaic or rigid, or a tool with elements to be completed or ticked off, like a to-do-list or as an assessment. Used properly with individuals, exploring ambivalence draws out, evokes, the most unexpected and unique information which can be startling to the owner and sometimes surprisingly emotional.

A template for exploring ambivalence is outlined, and this can be used collaboratively (4.10) with the owner to jot down their thoughts in the same way as was used with the scales and timeline in Chapter 7. A pre-printed template (see Chapter 14) can be used and kept handy for any opportunities to have conversations around ambivalence as they arise. The structure can just as easily be drawn out on a piece of paper. As the exploring ambivalence structure becomes familiar and integrated into your practice, it is possible to use the whole or just parts of the exploring ambivalence framework in conversation, keeping the structure in your head. This works well but takes a bit of time and practice to master.

Therefore, it is suggested that a paper template is used at first as, although this framework for exploring ambivalence looks very simple, it can be deceptive. Another reason to use a preprepared template is that when getting into the work with owners, anything that can help the worker to keep conversations structured and focused will be advantageous to both parties.

Those to whom we teach MI are often surprised about how tricky this innocuous-looking structure can be, causing some to ignore it and not use it. But exploring ambivalence, and therefore this structure, is a key element to working with behaviour change and using MI. It is suggested that, without exploring ambivalence, your conversations will be poorer and nowhere near as effective. Therefore, stick with it and practice with one or more willing friends before starting to use it with clients or owners. This could be seen as an invitation to you to make a change to your own practice as it will take a bit of thought and work!

It is worth mentioning that the use of the visual framework to record on is very helpful as owners can see what they have said. It allows some, as you are writing for them, time to consider and identify their pertinent issues. Giving a completed framework to the owner to take away can have an impact as many will later ponder further on the conversation, rather like percolating a good coffee: it takes time. Some people have even been known to pin their exploring ambivalence frameworks on their fridges, especially when exploring their own human health behaviours.

Exploring ambivalence can be used throughout the stages of change but will probably be most useful in precontemplation (3.3), contemplation (3.4), and to some extent in the preparation stage (3.5). As people move into the action stage (3.6), they are likely to have mostly resolved their ambivalence, but you may still find times when it can be useful to return to one of the exploring ambivalence elements.

The framework (adapted from Miller and Rollnick 2013) for exploring ambivalence is as follows.

Current behaviour or situation	
The good things about...	**The not-so-good things about...**

Possible New Behaviour / Changed Behaviour or situation	
The not-so-good things about...	**The good things about...**

8.3 The Structure of the Exploring Ambivalence Framework

This structure is straightforward once you get used to it, but it can be deceptive when we first start using it. Practice is really helpful with this tool.

A clear agenda, or focus (Chapter 6), for the conversation is important, just as it is with the other structures outlined in the previous chapter. Once the agenda is clear, the owner can be invited to think about the current behaviour and, using the top two boxes, explore what is good, and then not-so-good, about the current behaviour. Then, to move on to thinking about making the change and what would be the not-so-good and good things about that.

The exploring ambivalence framework needs to be introduced and the owner invited to discuss in more detail the identified behaviour. Undertake the whole process in a conversational manner and allow enough time. When done well, exploring ambivalence can be rich in detail and consequently may take more time than you might expect. The whole thing doesn't need to be done all at once though. Different elements can be discussed in different time slots.

Reset or reaffirm the agenda, perhaps saying something like,

Worker: *'Thinking about Sandy's diet, I wonder if you would be happy to explore that a little more with me... we would start by thinking about where you are now with his diet and how that works for you and then we would look at your thoughts about how changing his diet might be...'*

8.4 Current Behaviour / Situation

First, the owner is invited to talk through the current behaviour and what is good, or what works about it, and then what is not-so-good.

8.4.1 The Good Things about the Current Behaviour / Situation

Being asked about the good things about the current situation, the current behaviour, allows the owner to voice their sustain talk. It's there in their heads, so let's get it out and have a look at it!

> WORKER: *'Thinking about Sandy's diet... what are the good things about his diet at the moment / about how you feed him?'*

Owners will generally have some very good reasons for the behaviour and current situation (sustain talk 4.9). They need to get these out, and at the very least, the worker and the owner are clearer about the situation and the underpinning reasons for it.

However, often when the owner voices out loud the good things about a current behaviour (sustain talk 4.9), the reasons for it can sound a bit flat or lose their energy. When the worker, using all those active listening skills (Chapter 5), hears and accurately reflects back the sustain talk with neutrality (4.10.4), curiosity and kindness, owners often stop and say with surprise,

> *'There actually aren't that many good reasons when I really look at it.'*

Just asking about the current behaviour can be an amazing way to gain engagement and build a rapport with an owner. In the human health world someone who smokes may never have been asked about the good things for them about cigarettes, or for those who drink, the good things about alcohol. In past conversations, they may have had to argue with health professionals, using their sustain talk which probably was unheard. So, asking an owner this question and exploring further can really shift the dynamic and their experience in many ways.

If a paper template is being used, write down what the owner says as bullet points, using their own words and language as much as possible. What owners say may need to précised or shortened to brief points but these should be offered back to the owner to check they are correct before being committed to paper.

Once the owner has exhausted their reasons for the current behaviour, it is helpful to offer them a mini summary (5.17), to allow them to hear their words and reasons given back to them. The worker can ask the owner if they have any other thoughts about what is good about their current behaviour. One of the benefits of making bullet points to record the discussion is it can really help the worker to give very accurate and detailed mini summaries. For the owner, seeing their own words written down, as well as hearing accurate reflecting and summaries, can really change their perspective.

Box 8.1   Discussing What is Good About the Current Behaviour / Situation

When we are new to MI, it can seem counterintuitive to ask the owner to focus on what is good about the current behaviour or situation. We want, or even need, owners to change. We can worry about asking what is good about what they are doing right now. It can feel as if we are somehow encouraging them to stay the same, or are condoning the behaviour when we should be pushing for change or we should be fixing problems. Miller and Rollnick describe that fixing reflex (2.2.8) in which helpers or professionals can see what needs to be done and have the urge to get stuck in and make everything alright. The fixing reflex also fits with the traditional methods of behaviour change examined in Chapter 2, which generally just don't work! Therefore, asking and spending time exploring the good things or what works about the current behaviour can feel counterintuitive, tricky or uncomfortable for workers when using it for the first time.

8.4.2   The Not-So-Good Things about the Current Behaviour / Situation

When the good things about the current behaviour or situation have been exhausted, the worker moves on, asking the owner if they might explore the not-so-good things. Remember to be neutral (4.10.4) and work with kind curiosity. Possibly, in the past, others have told the owner what the problems are with their behaviour. If that has been the case, the owner is likely to have been so busy generating sustain talk (4.9) that they have never been able to voice the not-so-good things themself.

> 'And now thinking about the not-so-good things about not changing Sandy's current diet and the way you feed him... what would they be?'

The owner may start to verbalise some change talk (4.10.2). The worker should selectively reflect (5.16) what the owner is saying but also listen out for movement back and forth between change talk and sustain talk. Sometimes, owners will vacillate between the good and not-so-good things about the current behaviour. Any new information about the good things with the current behaviour can be added to the first box. The worker may have a role here to pull out which is which and clarify this with the owner.

As the owner considers what is not so good about the current behaviour, they may begin to mention the future, how it would be if things continue as they are. This can be useful for the worker to listen out for and then support the owner to explore. The timeline (7.3) asks the owner to look backwards, to how their current situation arose. Here, in exploring ambivalence there can be an opportunity for the owner to look forwards at a future with <u>no</u> behaviour change. If you think that it is appropriate and will not generate discord you could ask the owner something such as,

> 'If you look ahead and things don't change, they stay the same, how does the future look?'

Asking what is not so good about the current situation can be the start of evoking change talk (4.10.2), no matter how tentative. It can be hard for anyone to admit that their behaviour may not be the best. It can be even more difficult to admit this out loud to another person and one who may be a professional or even be in a position of authority. The worker's attitude will be key, keeping in mind the spirit of the approach of MI (4.5), ensuring they use a guiding style (5.12.3) and are listening well (5.8). The worker will need to be generous, gentle, and kind but confident in guiding and keeping the owner on track to the agreed agenda (Chapter 6).

Top active listening skills are essential (5.8), especially the use of reflecting (simple and complex 5.16). A mini summary (5.17) is again used at the end on this section and then the owner is asked if there is anything else they would like to add.

The worker needs to stay with what the owner gives them, even if something very obvious is omitted. When the glaringly obvious is not mentioned by an owner, resist leaping in and pointing it out to them. They may not know the same information as the worker, or it may be just too difficult, or shameful for them to say at that moment.

However, it is possible to offer information that the owner hasn't identified, when all four areas of the exploring ambivalence grid have been completed.

The worker should judge if offering something would be helpful and not cause the owner to increase sustain talk and back off. When information is offered (9.7), it should be done tentatively. An example of one way to do it might be,

> *'I have a thought about this, and I wonder if it would be helpful for me to share it...?'*

However, be cautious. Words should be chosen with care and offered cautiously. It is easy to get ahead of the owner here and lose the momentum towards change.

8.5 Changed Behaviour / Possible New Behaviour / Situation

Invite the owner to now think about how a behaviour change or a change to their situation might be. Be thoughtful about how you word this, neither leading the owner in any way nor having expectations of them.

8.5.1 The Not-So-Good Things About Changed Behaviour / Possible New Behaviour / Situation

Start with what would be not-so-good about a new or a different behaviour or situation. This area can bring more richness of information for both the owner and the worker. It can generate detail about what might get in the way of change for the owner, what might be difficult, what hasn't worked in the past. This can be valuable to use when the owner starts to move towards the preparation stage (3.5) of change or even for the action stage (3.6). Detail generated here can help identify potential difficulties, pitfalls, or experiences from past attempts to change. This evidence can be used to support the owner later if they decide to start setting goals (Chapter 10).

> *'Now, could you think about the not-so-good about changing Sandy's diet or changing how you feed him...?'*

Again, active listening should be used, reflecting (5.16) sustain talk (4.9) and change talk (4.10.2). Then, a mini summary (5.17) is offered by the worker and anything else the owner may think of can be added to this box, or to the others.

8.5.2 The Good Things About Changed Behaviour / Possible New Behaviour / Situation

Finally, the owner is invited to consider what might be good about a possible behaviour change or changing the situation.

> *'Now, might we look at what you think would be the good things about making a change to Sandy's diet / how you feed him?'*

Although it can be hard, it is essential for the worker to keep a neutral stance (4.10.4) here – it can be very easy to get excited when some change talk is heard and then to jump ahead of the owner. The owner is <u>not</u> being asked to make a change, rather just to ponder and think about what possible change might be like. The worker's whole approach needs to convey this via tone of voice, the pace, verbal and non-verbal body language (5.2–5.5) and carefully chosen words.

Change is tricky to think about. It can be difficult and stressful. The owner may need to backtrack and give reasons for not changing. It may look or feel so difficult that they may well give some more sustain talk. If this happens, the worker should acknowledge this sustain talk (4.9) and then pick up and reflect any change talk (remember dancing not wrestling 4.10.1). This is where double-sided reflecting (complex reflections 5.16.1.3) really come into their own as powerful tools. Double-sided reflections allow you to offer back to the owner both sides of the their ambivalence.

> '*On the one hand, you enjoy sharing good times and treats with Sandy as he is part of your family, and on the other, you see him putting on weight and you worry about his health, especially in the longer term.*'

A mini summary of this last box, the good things about possibly making change, can then be followed by an overall summary (5.17). Do this by going back over all the boxes in the order done, using the notes or bullet points in each. Although this can feel a bit repetitive for the worker, it can be enormously helpful to the owner to have their words and views fed back in different ways throughout the exploring ambivalence structure. The owner can then be invited to give feedback about what their thinking is now, perhaps by asking them,

> '*What do you make of that...?*' or '*What are your thoughts?*' or '*Where does this leave you now?*'

It is likely that the conversation will continue and a guiding style should be maintained (5.12.3) to keep what the owner voices to the agreed agenda. Retaining your spirit of the MI approach (4.5) with all its neutrality (4.10.4) and other underpinning principles will be essential. Throughout this exercise, you may hear importance and confidence (7.10) stated as feelings, thoughts, or beliefs from the owner. These are key to pick up and to explore. The importance and confidence scales (7.11) could be used or repeated, following the use of the exploring ambivalence framework.

Box 8.2   A Word on the Use of Words

The use of language in the exploring ambivalence framework is carefully thought out. You will notice the use of 'the good' and the 'not-so-good'. Using these words has been found in our training to come across as more neutral and so in keeping with spirit of the MI approach. For example, consider if the words 'good' and 'bad' were used - there would immediately be a bias, possibly prompting the owner to give answers they thought we or others wanted. Language, even single words, can make the owner feel that workers have their own agenda and this can lead to increased sustain talk, a reduction or absence of change talk, and the possibility that the owner will back away from the conversation.

Other unhelpful language to avoid are words and phrases such as 'pros' and 'cons' or 'benefits' and 'costs' or even a 'cost benefit analysis'. Many of us would run away if we were told to do a cost benefit analysis! Again, these words and phrases are weighted and are not neutral.

The use of 'the good' and 'the not-so-good' does make this harder for the worker though, as there often is a double negative in one of the boxes. This takes some thinking about and the worker needs to be clear about what it is that they are asking the owner. For example, when a behaviour change might be around neutering a companion animal, you might ask,

'What are the good things about not neutering your cat' and then the double negative of 'what are the not-so-good things about not neutering your cat.'

Once we have practiced and are confident, the double negatives are less of an issue and we can explain the process clearly to owners. However the need to become skilled and confident with the wording is one of the reasons that the exploring ambivalence framework is worth practicing with willing friends or colleagues before using it with your clients and owners.

8.6   Supporting Information for Using Exploring Ambivalence

Generally, aim to start with exploring the not-so-good things about the current behaviour and move through to finish at the good things about changing the behaviour. However, this may not always be possible. So long as the worker keeps a focus and structure to the conversation, hearing the owner's sustain talk (4.9) and evoking change talk (4.10.2) is the most important element.

It is possible that only the first one or two boxes might get done in a consultation or visit and the other areas can be explored at a later date. It is up to you, as the worker, about how to use this structure. Practice adapting to the owner, and undertake your own reflection-on-action (5.10) afterwards to consider what worked and how it might be used or done differently next time.

The owner may give the same or similar information for two different areas of the exploring ambivalence structure. You may also think that two areas will be the same. Not uncommonly, the same information and observations from the owners do occur in two boxes; however, it is highly likely that the meaning in one box will have a different meaning in another box.

For example, the good things about not changing may look very similar to the not-so-good things about change. Through the conversation and exploration you have with the owner, the same issue in each can have very different meanings in different places. An example of this is given below with someone who might need to reduce or stop breeding their animals.

Example – Current behaviour or situation – continuing to breed	
The good things about continuing to breed An income Gives me a focus Something to hand over to my kids Keeping the bloodline going Continuing the line I inherited from my father	**The not-so-good things about continuing to breed**
Possible new behaviour / changed behaviour / situation – reducing or stopping breeding	
The not-so-good things about reducing or stopping breeding Reduced income. What would I do with my time and energy? Who would I be if I didn't have this business? What would I leave to my kids? The end of the bloodline that my father and grandfather built up.	**The good things about reducing or stopping breeding**

These two boxes have very similar content but when explored, have very different meanings and give a fuller picture with two sides of the feelings and beliefs explored. This can elicit information about that person's frame of reference (Chapter 1), how they see the world, and how the behaviour fits into that.

When we add the information gained for the other areas in this example, we can see the ambivalence.

Example – Current behaviour or situation – continuing to breed	
The good things about continuing to breed	**The not-so-good things about continuing to breed**
An income	The market isn't there anymore for these animals.
Gives me a focus	
Something to hand over to my kids	It may never come back.
Keeping the bloodline going	I am struggling with the animals that I have especially now I am not selling so many and I am getting older.
Continuing that line I inherited from my father	
The market might come back, and I might make money again.	The kids aren't that interested and they may well not want the business, although I hope they will change their minds.
	It's costing more financially than I am making.
Possible change – reducing or stopping breeding	
The not-so-good things about reducing or stopping breeding	**The good things about reducing or stopping breeding**
Reduced income	I guess I will have to slow down or stop sometime, maybe now is the time to think about it.
What would I do with my time and energy?	
Who would I be if I didn't have this business?	I could reduce my costs.
What would I leave to my kids?	My worries would be less if I could sort out what I currently have and reduce the numbers.
The end of the bloodline that my father and grandfather built up	

With this example above, we can get a sense of the individual and their hopes and fears, beliefs, and concerns. There is some sustain talk (4.9) and some change talk (4.10.2). They are looking back to what they have done throughout their lives and also further back, to their father and grandfather. They are then looking forward to what the future might hold.

The final box – the good things about reducing or stopping breeding – actually has less in it. This is not uncommon, and as workers, there is the temptation to regard a longer list as better, as more indicative of change. However, it isn't about how long or short the list is in each box; it is about the meaning and impact for the individual.

8.7   Bear in Mind – This Is Not a Trick

Exploring ambivalence is not about tricking people into making changes. It is a framework to give structure to the conversations we have with owners and to allow them to voice sustain talk, have it acknowledged, and for change talk to be evoked.

While exploring ambivalence, your use of reflection-in-action (5.10) will be important to help you dance (4.10.1) with the owner as they move position and generate both sustain and change talk. A great deal can be learnt about the individual and their behaviour if this approach is used. Watch for the temptation to slide into the fixing reflex (2.2.8): that understandable human desire many, if not all, of us have to jump in and fix and make everything alright. Which doesn't work. Rather, there needs to be a focus on staying neutral (4.10.4) and not being tempted to argue in favour of change. Sometimes workers or others may try to manipulate the owner by arguing in favour of not changing in an attempt to force the owner into change (this is known as being 'paradoxical' and doesn't have a place in MI and behaviour change).

Box 8.3   Remember When Exploring Ambivalence

Ensure you and the owner both agree and are clear about the agenda/focus. As the worker, take time to draw out the grid in the order shown in the template.
    Use active listening.
    Watch for your own fixing reflex.
    Ask the owner to expand.
    Make it conversational in style.
    Be neutral.
    Ask the owner for feedback about how they found the conversation.

8.8   Exploring Ambivalence Can Be Emotional for the Owner

Be prepared for unexpected and unusual things to come to light. When anyone starts to weigh up the two sides, the different arguments for and against making a change, it can become uncomfortable. When ambivalence is experienced, a sense of discrepancy (4.8) often occurs in which values, beliefs, and goals are at odds with behaviour. This 'gap' (Clark et al. 2006) or sweet spot is the discrepancy between how people view themselves and what their behaviour is.

Experiencing discrepancy can be difficult. If people are to be helped to make change, they need support when feeling uncomfortable. There is a fine balance for the worker. If we help the owner feel really comfortable, they won't need to look at change, but if we generate too much discomfort, it becomes unhelpful to the owner. If there is too much discomfort, the owner can feel unable or unwilling to think about the change, consequently generate only sustain talk (4.9) with little or no change talk (4.10.2), back off from the conversation, disengage, and may even not return to work with us in the future.

I picture this discrepancy like receiving physiotherapy as a human. Physio can be darned uncomfortable and very hard work. It needs to have that sweet spot of enough work and discomfort to do its job, but not so much that it means we don't do any exercises or never return to our physio. Rather, a good physiotherapist will work with us, guide, and monitor what is manageable and the point when it becomes too much for us.

Box 8.4   Exercise

Find a willing colleague or friend.

Ask them if there is a health behaviour they would like to explore; it doesn't have to be one they definitely want to change, but one that they are happy to look at. Preferably an issue that is more a Ford Fiesta than a Ferrari one when practicing.

Starting a specific type of exercise or increasing exercise can be useful, as can altering a diet, eating less fat or sugar, for example, or more fibre or fruit and vegetables.

Set aside some time and ask them if they are willing to help you to develop your skills by talking about their chosen behaviour and for you to use a structure that you would like to practice (the exploring ambivalence framework).

Use the template (14.6) to guide you and before you start, work out what you are going to ask for the headings in each box; this will help to get things in the right order and also help with any double negatives. Remember, you may need to spend a little time being clear about the agenda and focus of the discussion rather than going for a broad subject such as 'I want to be happy!' or 'I want to be fitter'. And remember that the agenda or focus is not a goal – we are not asking people to set goals at this stage, although sometimes, people do come up with them for themselves, and if that is the case, use what they give you.

8.9   Using Exploring Ambivalence in Difficult Conversations

Once you become familiar with the exploring ambivalence structure or framework, you may find that it is an extraordinarily useful approach to use in difficult conversations. Examples from animal welfare colleagues are where exploring ambivalence is used to discuss giving up or signing animals over to a charity or another person. A number of my colleagues use it when they need to discuss euthanasia and report very good outcomes for the animal, the owner, as well as for them as worker. Other tricky conversations where it may be useful could be end-of-life discussions and one where there is a decision needed about continuing or stopping treatment.

8.10   Where to Next?

Where we go next after exploring ambivalence will depend upon where in the Stages of Change Model (Chapter 3) the individual is at that moment. You might want to look at the importance and confidence scales (7.10) and maybe, if appropriate, look at the readiness scale, or return to these scales. You might move to a typical day (7.6) if you haven't already done it or perhaps do a second typical day with creativity in how it is used. A timeline (7.3) or a return to the timeline may be appropriate. You will decide. You now have an increasing number of structures available for your conversations, as well as the Stages of Change Model, to help guide where you might go next in a conversation with an owner. Another technique which helps the owner to look forward can be found in the next chapter.

8.11   Conclusion

In this chapter, we have looked at one method for structuring conversations that helps to support people to explore their ambivalence about change. This structure – helping to guide an owner to explore and resolve ambivalence – is central to supporting behaviour change.

Using the tool is not as easy as it first looks, and it can be challenging for workers until they become comfortable with it. However, with some practice and experimentation, this can be the most useful structure you will use. I encourage you to work at using it until you become fluent and it fits easily into the conversations that you have.

Remember that the theories, ideas, and evidence-based methods presented and described in this book are not formulaic or linear. Rather, the concepts and techniques are to help workers listen, to support an owner to explore their situation, their unique experiences, perspectives, beliefs and feelings, and for them to be the ones to talk themselves into any changes they may make. Exploring and resolving ambivalence is the central component to what leads people to make changes.

References

Clark, M, Walters, S., Gingerich, R. and Meltzer, M. (2006) Motivational Interviewing for Probation Officer: Tipping the Balance toward Change. *Federal Probation.* 70, 1.

Miller, W. and Rollnick, S. (2013) *Motivational Interviewing: Helping People Change.* 3rd ed. New York: Guilford Press.

9

Supporting Preparation for Change – Envisaging Change

9.1 Introduction

The previous chapter looked at the importance of exploring ambivalence and introduced a framework to help structure conversations around this. Chapter 7 looked at the timeline (7.3) which gives us a way of helping the client or owner to see where they are and to look back at how they got there. Whilst exploring ambivalence with the owner you will often hear information about the past, elements that describe or help populate a timeline and understanding about how their current situation came about. Exploring ambivalence will also generate thoughts, beliefs, and feelings about the future. This will often give information about how the owner sees the future if they don't make changes, what it might be like if they did make a change, what would be difficult and what might be helpful if they made the change.

This chapter explores strategies to support people in the preparation stage of change, helping them to look ahead and envisage a change. It then covers ideas about how and when to offer people information and advice.

9.2 Preparation Stage of Change

In the Stages of Change Model (Chapter 3), contemplation with its ambivalence (3.4) comes before preparation (3.5). In the preparation stage, the person is moving towards making a change. Their ambivalence (3.4, 4.8) becomes more weighted towards the change end. People who are in preparation start to make plans even if these are merely tentative ideas. They begin to imagine what change might be like, they may look for information and ask questions of others. Preparation is an

Practical Human Behaviour Change for the Health and Welfare of Animals,
First Edition. Bronwen Williams.
© 2024 John Wiley & Sons Ltd. Published 2024 by John Wiley & Sons Ltd.
Companion website: www.wiley.com/go/williams/human

important stage, but it is often underestimated by both the person needing to make the change and those around them. What needs to be done in preparation is essential to setting a good foundation for a successful and sustained change.

As people move towards and into the preparation stage, they will generate less sustain talk (4.9) and more change talk (4.10.2). They may ask us, or others, questions about making the change, how to go about doing it, or what the change might be like once they get there.

You will also hear, in the owner's use of language, more resolve to make the change. For example, they may start to use wording such as 'I will', 'I need to', 'when I start making the change'. They will begin to imagine, to envisage, how the change might look and be for them. They may also start experimenting. An example of experimenting might be someone who smokes and, as they move into the preparation stage, changes brands, tries rolling their own or delaying their first cigarette to later in the day.

Similarly, an animal owner might start experimenting: buying different food for their animal, trying different routines. They may ask you or others for advice or perhaps look online or post questions on online forums, read about different ideas, approaches, or strategies for what they need to do. A dog owner for example, could start asking other people about where they walk their dogs, think about arranging to walk with another owner, even look at some maps of footpaths, or download an app on their phone to plan or record walks.

As people move towards, or just briefly dip a toe into the preparation stage of change, there are ways in which we can offer support to develop their thinking. One of these methods is to ask them to envisage hypothetically what a change might be like. A strategy called 'a look over the fence' can help with this.

Making a behaviour change is like undertaking a journey, perhaps a road trip. To drive to a destination, there needs to be some idea about where that end point is and the reasons for journeying there. There may be a vision of what it might look like upon arrival, even before the route planning stage, before the satnav is programmed. If we don't have a journey's end in mind, the purpose of it, it is very difficult to even begin to plan. It is similar with behaviour change: people need to be able to envisage the change, even if they don't decide to make it right now.

Working with those with substance use problems, drugs or alcohol, I was often struck by how difficult it was for them to envisage a successful change. They were so focused on the difficulties of making the change, of stopping substances, that often there were no ideas or no clear thoughts about being substance free and what that might be like. For those with substance misuse issues, other people repeatedly give their views of how change would be, but the individual usually lacks that vision for themselves. Those with addictions rarely know anyone who has made successful changes. Those who do stop drugs and alcohol usually choose, or need, to move away from old substance using friends and contacts, and they will often move locations and areas. Therefore, those still using substances generally lack role models to help them see that change is possible and that it can even be good! Many substance misuse services now employ people in recovery from their own substance problems as mentors, experts by experience, or peer workers to help others see that change is possible (see self-efficacy 11.15 and vicarious experiences 11.16.2).

Similarly, for those with animals, it may be difficult for them to envisage or imagine doing things differently; making a change. They may not know others who manage their animals in ways that are more welfare-friendly. Indeed, some owners may be surrounded by people. including family, friends and others who also manage their own animals in the same way. Outdated, inappropriate ways and / or poor welfare methods can be shared norms for some groups and communities (1.4.3). It can be difficult for owners of animals in these situations to envisage doing anything differently or to even realise there may be a problem or that there can be other ways of doing things.

Box 9.1   Exercise

Be on the lookout for a friend or colleague who talks about needing to make a change but is finding it difficult and is perhaps stuck. People often talk about difficulties around exercising, eating as healthily as one might, reducing scrolling on one's phone or even staying on top of chores, cleaning or sorting out possessions of theirs or those of a family member.

Listen out for how stuck that person may be. Notice if they describe how it is currently, but how difficult it is to implement changes and remedies. Notice if there is a lack of actually envisaging the change, seeing a change truly occurring, and how that would work for them.

9.3   Envisaging Change – A Hypothetical Look Over the Fence

A hypothetical look over the fence is another structure from MI that can support conversations around change. This hypothetical envisaging allows the owner to look ahead, to think about what a change might look like but without any pressure to have to make that change. It gives distance and freedom to think and explore, without the worries and concerns about change. A hypothetical change may be less threatening to consider than an actual change. It enables workers to have a conversation with an owner about the behaviour change without the individual feeling they are expected to make the change.

The approach to supporting hypothetical thinking about change is relatively simple, but like many of the MI methods, it can actually generate a lot of often surprising detail, discussion and thinking from the individual. To ensure that potential depth and richness can be elucidated by the owner, workers needs to take time, be curious, guide the person (5.12.3), use top-quality active listening (5.2–5.8), reflect specifics heard (5.16) and to ask about the details.

The worker simply asks the owner to think hypothetically about how it would be for them if they made a change in a behaviour or their situation. This can help the owner to further explore the importance of any change. The emphasis is on how things would be different if... there was hypothetically a change. It is easy to be weighed down with the anxiety, concerns, and issues that thoughts about making change often bring. These are the feelings and thoughts that can create sustain talk (4.9) for any of us, can paralyse or freeze us and prevent consideration of a change in a balanced way. Thinking hypothetically about making the change gives the freedom to envisage actually being successful. Many people who are stuck and unable to make changes don't have a vision of how the future might look with change, therefore much of what might be good about possible change is missed and instead there is focus upon the difficulties of change and how it might be easier to stay the same.

9.4 Inviting the Owner to Think Hypothetically About a Possible Change

How the worker introduces the hypothetical question will be key in how successful this structure is for the owner. Ensure that you are clear that the owner only needs to imagine how it might be, that they are not being asked to make the change. Allowing people to think hypothetically enables them to explore it freely and without stress and a lack of confidence that they may usually experience. It also helps to reduce sustain talk (4.9), generate change talk (4.10.2) and can give an owner a more positive idea of what might be possible.

For some people, the word 'hypothetical' may not be one that they understand, and different wording might need to be used to explain what it is that we are asking them to think about.

Support the owner by guiding (5.12.3) them to explore. Offer prompts to help them hypothetically consider the change in as much detail as possible. Often, the worker can ask a range of open questions (5.14) as well as selectively reflecting change talk (5.16.1.2). Listen for a move from sustain talk to increased change talk and anything that indicates increases in importance, confidence, and readiness (7.10) to make the change.

Box 9.2   Some Ways to Ask the Hypothetical Look Over the Fence Question...

'Can I ask you to imagine just for a moment, hypothetically... I'm not asking you to make the change, just imagine... If you had made the change... If you were looking over a fence and you could see yourself having made the change...'

- What would it be like, look like, feel like?
- What is most likely to have worked?
- How did it happen?

Other ways to help owners think about the change without feeling pressure

You could also ask,

- Imagine that a big obstacle has been removed – how might you be able to make the change?
- If you were to try to make the change again, what would you try?
- What would you tell someone else in your situation to do / what might help them?
- Imagine five years in the future from now and you had made the change. Looking back, what would you tell yourself now?

An example of a hypothetical look-over-the-fence conversation might be as follows:

WORKER: 'If you were to just think about an ideal situation for Sandy, looking over a fence into the future, I am not asking you to make the change but just to think about it hypothetically... if you had got him to his ideal weight... how might that be?'

OWNER: *'Well, you and other people would not be on my case anymore.'* [laughing]

WORKER: 'You would be having an easier time from people like me.' (reflecting)

OWNER: *'Yes, but also, you know, Sandy would be healthier and I guess happier. I would feel less worried about him... and you know, less bad about his health.'*

WORKER: 'Can you tell me a bit more about how that would be for you?' (open question)

OWNER: *'Well, it would be pretty nice now I think about it... I always have this nagging in the back of my head that I am doing him harm, but then I can't resist him wanting treats.'*

WORKER: 'Even when you feed him treats now, you have a worry at the back of your mind which is uncomfortable...Thinking again hypothetically about if things were different for you and Sandy, how would it be if that worry wasn't there anymore?' (reflecting then guiding back on track to the hypothetical question)

OWNER: *'Well, I could get on with other things and worry about those things!'* [laughs again] *'But seriously, I could really enjoy my time with Sandy and do more with him.'*

WORKER: 'What that would be like?' (open question to support envisaging)

OWNER: *'Well, we would be able to do longer walks, meet up with friends and family who have dogs, and do the walks that they do. Sandy and I would really enjoy that, both of us.'*

WORKER: 'Both you and Sandy would be able to get more enjoyable exercise and some increased socialising with people who might be important to you...' (reflecting)

OWNER: *'Yeah... You know, I hadn't really thought about all of that... but now we are talking about it, there is much more to this than just the titbits I feed Sandy...'*

9.5 Another Way of Supporting Envisaging – The Miracle Question

A very similar technique, from a different intervention for helping people called solution-focused therapy, asks the individual to imagine that while they are asleep, a miracle happens overnight. This miracle creates changes and their problem or issue is resolved, but the person is unaware that this has happened. The person is asked if they woke up one morning and the miracle had materialised without their knowledge, what would be the first thing they would notice, would see, hear, feel, and so on. We might ask the person about how they would behave, what they would do, and also how others would behave and respond to them.

Box 9.3   Exercise

If you have any children in your life, perhaps try out the miracle question with them when they have a problem or a worry. Kids can be great to practice with as they often really engage with this and are brilliant at using their imagination. Have fun with it and see what they teach you about how hypothetical / envisaging can work.

The questions, from the miracle question, about senses and feelings, can be asked within the hypothetical look over the fence strategy. Or, for some people the miracle question may be easier for them to work with. With a little practice you will be able to decide how you use these ideas to support your owners to envisage change.

Box 9.4   Example of a Hypothetical Look Over the Fence

Some people respond really well to the visualising element of the hypothetical look over the fence. On one NHS course I taught many years ago, a young professional was one of the students and throughout the course, during the practice sessions with other students, she discussed her desire to have a car and to pass her driving test. This particular group were from a rural county and decided to call this exercise a 'look over the hedge' instead of 'over the fence'. During one of the final days of the course, the group practiced hypothetical envisaging with each other about how the change might be or could be. It was this exercise that had a huge impact on the young student. She reported back that when she was asked to think hypothetically about driving and what it might be like, she suddenly, for the first time, could imagine herself driving without anxiety. She said she imagined all of the anxiety being caught up in the hedge and on the other side of it she was free to drive without angst. Up until that point, she had never realised that it might be possible for her to drive and to not have anxiety! A number of years later, I received an email from her, saying that she had moved to a large city and was happily driving there. This example highlights that when people can be supported to free themselves from the burdens of concerns about change, they can see a very different future. This can be very helpful in supporting the building of confidence to make a change and the ability to envisage that change.

Box 9.5   Exercise

Find a willing friend, family member, or colleague who would be happy to talk about a behaviour they might want to consider changing. Practice using the hypothetical look over the fence.

Remember that you will need to explain that you are not asking them to make the change but rather, just for them to think hypothetically about how it might be if they made the change.

Remember to use your active listening, acknowledge and reflect sustain talk and especially change talk. Watch for and reflect any changes in importance, confidence and readiness.

> *Remember to spend time and allow them to explore how the change could be. You might want to use prompts around how it might feel, look, and so on. You could also ask how they and / or others could be impacted, what this would mean and perhaps what others would notice, feel, and say or do.*
>
> *Be prepared for surprises as, like many of the other techniques, all sorts of things can come to light during these conversations that will be unusual and unique to the individual, often surprising them as well as us. These surprises and revelations are some of the joys of working with people exploring possible behaviour changes and bring richness and diversity to our work to keep us, as workers, interested and on our toes!*

9.6 Asking the Owner What Advice They Would Give to Someone Else

Another technique that can be useful to help someone get a little distance from their sustain talk and worries about the difficulties of change can be to ask them how they might advise someone else in a similar situation.

This is often a very quick and simple but effective technique. Ask the person to pause and then think about if they were to advise someone with a problem or behaviour change such as theirs, what would they say? As discussed in Chapter 2 (2.2.2), we all like to give advice to others about what they need to do and what would be best for them. So, we can harness this and ask the owner for the advice they would give someone else. This way they get advice from the expert on their situation – themselves!

Box 9.6   Exercise

Look out for opportunities to ask someone, when they are struggling with a dilemma, a problem or a behaviour change, what advice they would give to someone else in a similar position. This can be extremely useful if you have children as they respond really well to this. Try out this quick technique and see what happens!

9.7 Giving Information

Up until now, it has been suggested that we avoid wherever possible giving information. If you remember, in the traditional approaches to behaviour change (Chapter 2) (which generally don't work), we tend to tell, inform, advise, and give leaflets and information.

Giving information is a very important element of animal health and welfare work, but the knack is knowing when and how to do it. Pitching information at the wrong time, in an unsuitable way, or without understanding the owner's perspective will make things worse, not better. When used unhelpfully, the giving of information can damage engagement with an owner. It can cause the person to withdraw from the conversation or from the working relationship with us and to even be less likely to engage with others who might help them in the future. Unwise or untimely information giving can be a driving factor for discord (3.8, 4.6) between the worker and the owner and, even worse, can generate sustain talk (4.9) with little or no change talk (4.10.2) and so harden the individual into the behaviours they are currently doing, or not doing. Giving information at the wrong time or in the wrong way can actually make change less likely.

So, how can we give information when it can be received and be helpful to the individual?

First, consider what you are hearing from the owner and where they might be, at that moment, in the stages of change. If you have a sense that they are currently in the preparation stage (3.5), it may be appropriate to give information, but only if the individual wants it and can find useful.

9.8 Ask-Offer-Ask

MI gives a very simple framework to deliver information in a really supportive way, called 'ask-offer-ask' (Miller and Rollnick 2023).

Ask: First, ask if the owner might like some information. If they say yes, ask what they already know, then what specifically they would like information about. This allows us to tailor the information to what the owner requires, asks for, or is ready to hear. When giving information, it is easy to leap in and give everything that we think needs to be delivered. Often, people already have a level of knowledge. In fact they may already be well informed and are often the experts in their own behaviours (4.7.2). For example, people who smoke, when asked what they know about smoking generally have a great deal of knowledge and almost as much as, sometimes more than, the human health workers trying to educate them.

Even if animal owners have less knowledge than workers, they are still the experts on their lives, their situation, and their frame of reference on the world and their animals (Chapter 1).

By asking, workers can then sometimes hear incorrect information that the owner believes or which is now out of date as the evidence base has moved on, or myths they may have been told, or which are held by their community or culture. An example might be an owner telling you that cats can't get pregnant by their siblings.

Offer: The requested information is offered. This is tailored to what the worker knows about the owner, the relationship with them, and most importantly, to what information they have requested. It is vital that the worker keeps a neutral stance (4.10.4) and avoids adding in a few flourishes or facts to try and persuade or even scare the owner.

Ask: Lastly, the worker asks what the owner makes of the information provided, if it was useful, how it fits with what they think, know, and believe. The owner may ask more questions at this point, and the worker can identify anything that may have been misunderstood or is not sufficiently clear.

It might sound like this:

WORKER: 'When we talked about you looking over the fence and seeing how things might be with Sandy and his weight, you had some interesting thoughts about that. I wonder if there is any information you need from me at all about weight and diet for dogs?' (ask)

CLIENT: *'Well, one thing I was wondering about was...I have seen these different types of food for dogs with different issues; there is information in your waiting room.'*

WORKER: 'You have seen some information about different feeds available for dogs. What would be useful for you to know right now?' (simple reflection followed by ask)

CLIENT: *'Well, I'd like to know more about what a special diet like those advertised might do for Sandy and his weight. I had always thought they were an expensive luxury, but I guess I would really like to know if they work. Would I be better looking at a diet like that for Sandy or looking at what I already feed him and reducing that?'*

WORKER: 'You would like to understand more about the specialised diets for you to be able to weigh up what the next step for you and Sandy might be about his diet – is that right?' (reflecting to clarify)

CLIENT: *'Yes, please.'*

WORKER: 'Well, there are specific diets available for dogs who need to lose weight. There is a veterinary nurse who is specially trained in giving advice about diets, and she could help you work out what would be the best food for Sandy and what target weight to aim for. Many of the dry foods come with measuring scoops; so, although the food can appear expensive, if you follow the diet and measure correctly, you could find it wasn't as costly as you might have thought.' (offer)

CLIENT: *'Ok, that kind of makes sense.'*
WORKER: 'What do you make of this?' (ask)
CLIENT: *'I had been thinking about the cost I guess rather than actually how much to specifically give a dog. If the nurse was able to talk to me about it and work out what might work for Sandy, then I could understand the cost.'*

9.9   Offering Information – Asking to Be Invited

Sometimes, there is a key bit of information we think very relevant, but have held back from giving it to the owner as they have not specifically asked for it. If this is the case, then we can make an offer, or ask permission (Miller and Rollnick 2023) such as that below:

'There is a little more information that I am aware of, and although you did not ask about this, I wonder if you would find it useful if I shared it with you?'

Or, with Sandy's owner, it might sound like this:

WORKER: 'We can certainly look at an appointment for you and Sandy with the veterinary nurse who can talk to you about diets, if that is something you decide you would like to do.' (emphasising personal choice and responsibility) 'I do have another thought and wonder it it may be useful for me to share this with you?' (offering information that hasn't been asked for).
CLIENT: *'Go on...'*
WORKER: Well, some owners have found it useful to keep a kind of food diary for their dog for a week or so, writing down everything they give their dog, including regular food and any treats or titbits. It sometimes helps people to see how much their dog is eating over a period of time, and also, it can be useful for the first appointment with the nurse to discuss diet.'
WORKER: (after a pause) 'Does that sound like something that might work for you?'

When workers offer, ask to be invited or ask for permission, to give some information in this manner instead of leaping in and giving it when it is unsolicited, and if the relationship is working, people don't say no! This is a very respectful way of working that doesn't put pressure on an owner and is less likely to produce sustain talk (4.9) from them, or discord (3.8) in the relationship. It feels much more as if we are just putting the information on the table for us both to consider and discuss.

Box 9.7   Asking to Be Invited

I think of offering information rather like popping around to someone's house uninvited. We hover tentatively at the door and see if they might invite us in; we are offering them our company. We may or may not be asked in, but one thing we probably don't do is to stick a foot in the door as soon as they open it and elbow our way in. Offering information needs to be done in a similar way. Offering unsolicited information can be like kicking down someone's front door when we decide to visit them!

Some years ago, when I had a human health check up with my practice nurse, she asked if I wanted to know my BMI. I said yes, with a wince: I knew enough to expect it to be high. She gave me the number (which was high) and gave me some seconds to absorb that, and then we moved on. That part of the conversation stayed in my head for a number of months, if not a year due to the neutral and simple way it was given. I went on to change my lifestyle and lose weight, some stones; that tiny bit of information that was offered to me and how it was done was one of the elements that influenced me to make the change.

When information is being given, the worker will do more of the actual talking, but there still needs to be attentive listening to what the owner wants and the sense they make of the information given. There is a big temptation to jump in and resort to those traditional methods (that we know don't work, like kicking down the door) of telling, advising, informing, or trying to educate the person into submission (Chapter 2). We can get excited and caught up in the desire for the person to make a change especially when we see that this could be likely. The fixing reflex (2.2.8) that Miller and Rollnick talk about can loom large here; the worker can desperately want to help the person make changes, to do what seems obvious, even simple and which is in theirs or their animals' best interests.

As much caution needs to be exercised by the worker, when an owner is moving into the preparation (3.5) or action (3.6) stages of change, as is used for the precontemplation (3.3) or contemplation (3.4) stages. It is easy to overwhelm owners, for discord (3.8) to be created, for them to move away from the change, perhaps moving back in the stages of change to contemplation or precontemplation and even to disengage from workers or the agency or organisation.

Box 9.8   An Animal Analogy

An animal analogy may be useful here. Think about when you are working with one of your own animals, now or in the past. You are trying to either teach them something or to get them to trust you. When we work with animals and sense them relaxing with us, we still have to proceed cautiously. It would be easy to get carried away, go too fast at this point and for the animals to back off. And so it is with humans.

Box 9.9   Giving Tailored Information

When I ask my vet about end of life for one of my animals and how we can plan and manage it, I want very specific information tailored to my existing knowledge and which will add to it. With a subject like this, being given too much information that I already know, or haven't asked for, will be overwhelming, possibly upsetting and can stop me from hearing and absorbing what I do want and need.

It can be useful to remember the ideas of 'direct, follow, guide' (5.12). Some people will come just wanting the information, and a directing style (5.12.1) from us, and when this is the case, we can still use ask-offer-ask. At the very least, in these types of situations, it can save a whole load of time and energy in not giving superfluous information.

Box 9.10   Exercise

You might like to practice ask-offer-ask the next time you need to give someone any information. Be conscious of using this simple but effective framework; see how it goes when you stick to it and perhaps ask the individual for feedback about how they experienced it.

9.10   Conclusion

This chapter looked at ways to help people in the preparation stage of change to envisage or hypothetically look at the changes they might make. It then covered how information can be given when it is warranted and when the owner wants it.

The next chapter will continue to look at how to support people in the preparation stage for change, including how to help set goals and plans for action.

Reference

Miller, W. R., and Rollnick, S. (2023). *Motivational Interviewing: Helping People Change and Grow*, 4th ed. New York: The Guilford Press.

10

Preparation – Setting Goals, Making Action Plans and Contingency Plans

10.1 Introduction

The previous chapter described methods to support the preparation stage of change, including using hypothetical questions to help owners to envisage change and how information might be offered using ask-offer-ask. This chapter continues to look at how to support those in the preparation stage. It then covers strategies to help people prepare to move into action, including goal setting, action planning, and thinking about contingencies when things don't quite go to plan.

10.2 Goals

When using the traditional methods (Chapter 2) to try and make people change behaviour, the first thing we tend to do is to ask them about goals. We may go further and set the goals for them saying,

> 'So what you need to do is...'

It is easy to assume, without clarifying, what the owner needs, wants to do and what their goals are, and then we can head off in completely the wrong direction.

You will notice that in this book, goals come way after most of the other information, strategies and ideas. This reflects how goals generally come later in an owner's journey through the stages of change (Chapter 3).

Practical Human Behaviour Change for the Health and Welfare of Animals,
First Edition. Bronwen Williams.
© 2024 John Wiley & Sons Ltd. Published 2024 by John Wiley & Sons Ltd.
Companion website: www.wiley.com/go/williams/human

10.3 Goals Are Different to Agendas

Agendas (Chapter 6) come early in this book, goals much later. Agendas give workers and owners a shared understanding and agreement of what both are there for, the focus of conversations and what will be considered.

Owners may make goal statements in a number of the stages of change. In contemplation (3.4), these may be more of a statement of a wish or a desire for things to be different but without any real intent or perhaps ability to work towards those goals at that time. An example might be that I want to win the national lottery, but that is merely a wish and is far from a realistic or concrete goal as I almost never buy lottery tickets. When someone makes a statement that sounds like a goal, it is very easy for others to get excited and enthusiastic. We can wrongly assume the owner is ready to change right now, this minute, is fully committed to taking action and that they possess all the skills and things needed to make the change. When workers excitedly, but wrongly, assume a change is imminent they hear something very different to what the owner actually means. Agendas become mismatched (6.7), the worker's approach is not appropriate for the individual and the stage of change they are at that moment. A worker can easily tip into the fixing reflex (2.2.8) with a well-meaning desire for things to be well for the owner, and their animals, leading to a shift back to the use of traditional methods (Chapter 2). It may be useful to revisit Chapter 6 and the section on agendas as a reminder, especially the agenda matrix (6.7) which outlines how workers and owners can have matching or mismatched agendas.

However, statements of goals in the preparation stage (3.5) are likely to be different. Here, the owner has increasing intent to make a change and that change is likely to be more imminent. When owners are in the preparation stage, workers can help the person develop appropriate goals for both themselves and their animals and to define these goals more clearly.

So, agendas need to be identified, considered, negotiated, and set early in the process in working with someone around behaviour change. Goals generally come later, when the individual is further along in the stages of change.

10.4 Goal Setting

When people are moving into the preparation stage, not only is it is useful to start supporting them to think about goals but workers can help them to identify actions needed to get to these goals and also what might hinder them.

Take a few moments to reflect on the traditional approach to supporting people to make behaviour changes (Chapter 2). Often, the first thing that happens, as helpers try and promote behaviour change for someone, is that they immediately start to ask the person to think about setting goals, or worse, they start to set goals or targets for the person! This can be the easiest way to produce discord (3.8) within the working relationship. Rather, it is *evocation* (4.10.2) that is needed, to pull out of the individual how *they* would like to proceed towards any changes *they* might decide to make (emphasising personal choice and responsibility 4.10.4).

A criticism often made of goal setting for behaviour change is that not enough time is taken in developing goals. Problems occur when goals are not made specifically *with* the individual, or are made *for* the person by others. Goals need to be person-centred (4.10.1); relevant to, and driven and designed by the person incorporating their own expertise (4.7.2). Goals also need to be appropriate for the individual at that particular time or for their current position in life. Sometimes, workers may co-design goals and action plans with the client or owner where appropriate, preferably when invited to do so.

Other problems with goal setting are when they are generic rather than tailored to the individual, and either too simple or too complex. Often, there is little or no attention to how the person will work towards the goals, and this is where action planning (10.9) is key.

Box 10.1   The Importance of Action Plans

I often think of goals and action planning like a sandwich. Goals are the bread which hold it all together, but the action plans are the filling. Without the filling, there is no sandwich: it's just bread.

Box 10.2   Not Everyone Has the Skills that You Have!

Many of us working in professional roles have learnt pretty robust methods for setting goals and planning for action. You may, like me, love a good list, a plan, and perhaps have a notebook (or two) with you at all times. Our jobs, and maybe our backgrounds, have supported us to develop good planning and problem-solving skills. We have probably learnt these skills along the way and may have taken courses and seminars. Therefore, much of what is in this chapter may seem obvious. However, it is worth remembering not everyone has such well-developed planning skills. Some may have had them, but find them diminished due to cognitive changes, perhaps due to ageing, disease, or a brain injury. Others didn't have the support in their formative years (1.4.3) to develop robust skills needed for planning and goal setting. Others may be great at managing in one part of their lives but not in another, not realising that the skills they have can transfer across to animal ownership and care.

An example of this lack of expected basic knowledge and skills came from a story by a social care family worker. She described how she'd shown two young parents how to use a toilet brush to clean their toilet. This may sound extraordinary, but think about it – if you have never been shown how to use a toilet brush, never seen one used, how would you know?

As outlined in the previous chapters, workers need to support owners and others to understand, explore, and voice their beliefs about behaviours and their concerns about change. Hopefully, it now makes more sense why, when people are in the precontemplation (3.3) or the contemplation (3.4) stages of change, goal setting isn't appropriate. Their focus and perspective at that time probably won't support the formulation of goals. But, as an owner starts to indicate a willingness to consider change, as demonstrated through increased change talk (4.10.2) and reduced sustain talk (4.9), it can be the time to ask and explore what goals they might set.

As suggested in Chapter 9 and the hypothetical look over the fence (9.3), change is like a journey with an end point in mind. Having that vision of the end of the journey will be essential, whether physically travelling, or planning an expedition of behaviour change. Once that arrival point is identified and envisaged, planning can be started as to how to get there. When planning a physical trip, this can be the required steps or stages in the journey, the timeframes needed or available, what might help (a co-driver, someone to read the map, some sandwiches and coffee to take with you, money for tolls, filling up with fuel beforehand) and also what might hinder (rush hour, road or rail works, weather, the state of the vehicle, human tiredness) and how these things can be handled when they occur.

Therefore, the setting of goals, developing action plans and contingency plans is very similar to planning for a physical journey. Let's start to look at these elements in a bit more detail.

10.5 Goals and How to Support People to Formulate Them

Goals for behaviour change should be set by the individual, not workers or others. When appropriate, we can assist an owner to goal set and we can offer or be invited to help, but we should not force ideas upon them.

An owner's goal may appear to be unrealistic but they may need try it out and realise for themselves that it won't work. The worker can then assist an owner to review, reappraise, and reset the goal or the action plan with the new information gained. Often, owners see this as a failure, as can workers. However, something not working out as planned provides excellent information to aid understanding and to help avoid problems or issues that may trip the person up in the future. Few of us successfully make changes that stick at first attempt (3.9). Often we have to experiment, try out, and find what does and doesn't work for us. It may also be possible that as worker, our assumptions are incorrect and the person's goal and action plan works for them! After all, people are the experts (4.7.2) on their own lives and behaviours.

However, it is possible by using good listening skills (5.11) and the spirit (4.5) and structures of MI to help an owner assess their goal before finalising it. Considering a goal in depth allows re-evaluation and refining of goals before action is actually attempted. Timelines (7.3) can give some really helpful information here. They can be returned to and reviewed if previously undertaken, or can be used now for the first time. Timelines can generate practical details about what has and hasn't worked in the past and what has previously tripped the person up and therefore may do so again.

There are some ways workers can help owners to set and remodel their goals. Using a guiding style (5.12.3), workers can ask about the details of the goal, how it will work, and what actions are needed. Often, people will come to the conclusion that they need to amend or change their goal. The MI approach can continue to support people as they move to the preparation (3.5) and action (3.6) stages of change through guiding (5.12.3), active listening and in particular reflecting (5.16), asking open questions (5.14) and being neutral (4.10.4) whilst remaining curious.

10.6 Break Goals Down

As we know, behaviour changes can be overwhelming, and often, when we are working with animal owners, there may be big changes that need to be made overall. If possible, workers can support the owner by suggesting that large goals might be broken down into smaller ones. Then owners can be asked which would be the easiest or most important to start with. If people can start to experience a sense of achievement (11.16), it will help their self-efficacy or the belief that they can make change (11.15). This then supports their confidence and the ability to make other changes.

Box 10.3   Breaking Goals Down

Do you remember learning to tie your shoelaces as a kid? Initially, tying them was probably broken down into a serious of stages. I'm pretty sure it took a good number of attempts and experimentation to tie them in the way that you do now – probably with frustrations along the way and perhaps the short-lived decision to never bother with shoes again. This may remind us that skills need to be broken down into smaller elements and practiced until they become routine.

Box 10.4   SMART Goals

You may well have come across SMART as a mnemonic acronym for setting goals. SMART gives the specifics for goals that then are more likely to appropriate. We can share this with owners, and some may have come across it before, perhaps in their work settings. This allows owners to question their goals themselves without queries coming from the worker; rather, they come from applying the simple SMART model. Therefore, this can be more acceptable to the owner and less likely to create sustain talk or discord.

S – specific. Is the goal specific, is it is clearly outlined and not vague or ambiguous?

M – measurable. Can the individual identify when and how they plan to achieve their goal? If goals lack a measurable element the owner is less likely to experience a feeling of success or achievement. When these are lacking it can reduce their drive to change or continue. We all like to feel that we are succeeding. Change is hard work, and if we can't identify outcomes obtained for that effort, we can just give up and stop.

A – achievable. Is the goal just that – achievable for this person with the resources they have and the time frame they set?

R – realistic. Is the goal realistic and therefore achievable? We can ask the owner, 'How realistic is that goal for you right now?' Often, stated goals can be broad or wishful, like my desire to win the lottery but without my purchasing any tickets. Goals may need to be worked on and honed down to become realistic.

T – timed / timely. This element can be two things.

The first, *timed*, means – is there a timeframe for the goal? If there is this will help with focus, with reviewing progress, as well assisting action planning

The second, *timely*, means – is this goal appropriate for the time period identified – thus helping it to be realistic? For example, an owner might set a goal of feeding their horses more hay in the winter. However, if they were discussing it in the spring and the grass was coming through, it may not be a timely goal.

10.7 Developing Action Planning and Contingency Plans

Prompts can be used to assist the owner to explore their goals and their methods to achieve these, the actions needed, and also to be aware of what might get in the way (see 10.12). Rather than a list of questions to run through with the owner, these prompts are used to stimulate and open up conversations around the change and aid exploration. They will need to be adapted to the worker's personal style and the needs of the individual owner.

Box 10.5   Using Timelines and Scales to Support Plans

You may find that conversations around goals allow you to revisit structures and strategies already used earlier in the stages of change, including the scaling questions to explore importance, confidence, and readiness (7.10). A new timeline (7.3), or revisiting a timeline, can be especially useful here to allow people to consider what has helped and hindered in the past when they have made this, or other behaviour changes.

10.8   Using Avoidance Initially and Then Using Exposure

Some people may initially need to factor in or plan to avoid some situations which could trip them up and cause a return to an old behaviour. Once people become more confident, they can reintroduce those situations.

Think of someone who stops smoking and may well need to *avoid* their smoking friends and to side-step shops from which they used to regularly buy tobacco. They may need to remove ashtrays, lighters, and other smoking paraphernalia. Over time, contact with others and situations can be reintroduced as cravings, urges, and cues become more manageable.

Perhaps, for an animal owner who overfeeds, they might initially use *avoidance* by not having certain foods or snacks in the house or giving away those that they still have. Owners who have too many animals and need to stop taking on more may need to *avoid* social media and delete the associated apps for the time being, to prevent them seeing stories about and requests for homes for animals. These are just examples of avoiding and then reintroducing exposure to certain situations or experiences; each individual will be different and will need to explore and develop their own.

10.9   Action Planning

Action planning is a key part of behaviour change but is often missed out or glossed over. Goals can be seen as the 'what' needs to be done, but action planning is the 'how' to do it. A bit like that idea of preparing for a journey to travel somewhere. The goal would perhaps be our destination, but the action plan would be how the journey will be undertaken. A journey may be broken down into smaller goals with a number of stops that lead to the final goal destination.

Each of these stages may have an action plan. This may seem obvious but it is worth remembering that, although we may have well-developed skills and therefore could assume that everyone will have similar skills and abilities, many people do not. Some may be stressed, overwhelmed, or have other life difficulties at the point that they find themselves discussing a change in behaviour for the sake of their animals. Others may never have had the support and opportunities to develop good planning skills.

A little reminding or prompting here from the worker may be very useful and a basic template, like the one below, can help an owner frame their goal and an action plan to support it.

Goal	Action plan	Timescales	Who can help?

Writing information down to support the person to remember what they have identified can be helpful. Documenting assists people to stay on track and also to experience a sense of achievement. This can create energy that helps the individual persevere with their behaviour change and can also support self-efficacy. Section 11.15 has more information on self-efficacy and 11.16 on how to increase it.

The example below uses the template for the owner's goal and action plan where their animal needs to lose weight.

Goal	Action plan	Timescales	Who can help?
Date:			
Sandy to reduce 6 kgs of weight over four months	To record all of Sandy's food	Start today and continue daily	Family
	To book and attend appointment with nurse regarding diet	Next week	Veterinary nurse
	To decide on diet that will suit Sandy and owners for weight loss	Next week	Owner and nurse
	Weigh at surgery every two weeks with veterinary nurse	Biweekly	Owner and nurse
	Review with vet	In two months	Owner and vet

10.10   Contingency Plans

Contingency plans support people to stay on track when something threatens to disrupt plans or to challenge progress. Perhaps think of a behaviour you have changed in the past. Now think about some of the things that caused you to waver or not continue with the goal that you wanted to achieve. We can easily predict some of the things that will trip us up and contingency plans can be put in place to mitigate these in the future. Other, unexpected issues can catch us off guard, and this is why regular reviews of progress with owners can help. These experiences, and the subsequent knowledge generated, can support plans for future issues.

Again, a timeline (7.3) can be helpful here, done for the first time, or revisited, as it may well help the person to pinpoint issues or patterns from the past that have tripped them up. A timeline can also help identify the times problems have been successfully circumnavigated. Recalling past success can help with self-efficacy and so be helpful for making successful behaviour changes.

Contingency plans may appear to be just common sense. However, remember that not everyone has sufficient skills, experiences, and resources, and even if someone does have these, they can be hard to tap into when under stress or in difficulty. A plan or an outline can be incredibly helpful for when the unexpected happens.

Box 10.6   Exercise

Spend a few minutes drawing out a timeline for a change you have made in the past, even if you have gone back to the behaviour, perhaps many times. Diet or exercise may be one to think as these are changes most of us have attempted more than once. Or choose something else that is pertinent to you.

At first, just write down the times you made the changes and when.

Then, run through the timeline again and note what helped you make the change and then to keep going with it. Did anyone help you? What was happening in your life at the time, such as family, career, environment or something else? Did any of these things help you make a change?

Now, revisit the timeline and note down anything that tripped you up. What were these? When did they happen?

Notice, as you write these things down, if more information or patterns come to light.

A template for writing down a contingency plan is below.

Goal	What might get in the way of your goal and action plan?	When? How?	Contingency plan

Here is an example of perhaps what Sandy's owner's contingency plan might start with.

Goal	What might get in the way of your goal and action plan?	When? How?	Contingency plan
Sandy to reduce 6 kgs of weight over four months.	Sandy begging for food.	Mainly when we are eating a meal, and I feel sorry for him missing out.	Have a routine that Sandy is shut out of the living room when we are eating. Give him his favourite toy to distract him when he is shut out of the living room. Remind myself that we are doing this for his well-being and health. Make sure we give him play time after a meal and ask the rest of the family to help with this.

10.11 Questions to Support Conversations Around Planning Change

Below are some questions that workers might adapt to their own style, nature of the work, and the owner they are helping. They can help prompt conversations around goals, action planning, and contingency plans. These questions are not a script or a check list, rather they are suggestions to help frame conversations with an owner in the preparation stage of change (3.5). These questions can be very helpful to put the owner centre stage, making them the expert (4.7.2) on the situation and drawing upon their expertise.

Box 10.7   Top Tips
These questions need to be conversational, not tick list. Use them to help structure and open up the conversation. Remember to continue to use active listening (Chapter 5) and a guiding style (5.12.3). Don't underestimate ambivalence (3.4, 4.8) so watch out for an owner or client slipping back for a few minutes to contemplation stage (3.4). Watch for the person moving back and forth between preparation (3.5) and contemplation (3.4). Watch out for losing your owner if you misjudge their ambivalence causing them to back off, or for discord being generated (3.8).

10.11.1   What Might Be the Small First Step Towards Your Goal?

This can help the person to start to break down their goal into smaller, more achievable elements as well as to help them envisage (9.3) beginning the change.

Box 10.8   Example for Not Underestimating Ambivalence When Someone Is Considering Action

Imagine you have agreed to do a bungee jump... It seemed like a good idea... But now they are strapping you into the harness...you may now be thinking this was actually a really bad idea. This perhaps gives a sense of how people may make a decision, and then, as it gets closer to action, they back off or wonder if it is the right thing to do just at this moment...

10.11.2   What Might Get in the Way of You Working Towards Achieving This Goal?

This question invites the person to consider potential pitfalls and to begin to develop contingency plans if those snags occur. Revisiting a timeline (7.3) here may help identify issues from previous experiences that could reoccur.

10.11.3   How Do You Think You Can Overcome These Pitfalls?

Here you are asking the person to identify strategies themselves about how to overcome potential pitfalls. Again, the timeline may give clues as to what they have used successfully in the past. This can help with confidence for the change, their self-efficacy (11.15) and in developing a contingency plan.

10.11.4   What Methods Have You Found Helpful in the Past to Achieve This or Other Goals?

Asking this can help with self-efficacy (11.15) and the building of confidence by reminding the person of changes they have previously achieved and what they might use again and add to their contingency plan. Again, the timeline (7.3) may give clues if the person needs help to structure their ideas and thoughts.

10.11.5 What Is the Most Realistic / Easily Achievable of These Solutions?

Here you are supporting the person to structure and prioritise solutions in the action plan.

10.11.6 What Do You Think You Can Realistically Do By ...?

This question invites the person to return to the goal, to chunk it down into smaller elements, allowing a SMART goal (Box 10.4) and an action plan to be drawn up. However, be careful when asking this question: use a guiding style (5.12.3) and listen for any shift in direction away from preparation (3.5). It would be very normal to hear people vacillate between contemplation (3.4) and preparation (3.5) by expressing ambivalence (Chapter 8) with increases in sustain talk (4.9) and a reduction in change talk (4.10.2). By hearing and acknowledging the sustain talk, then evoking (4.10.2) change talk and reflecting this (5.16), workers can help an owner refocus. Be reflexive (5.9), dance with the owner (4.10.1) and shift position with them.

10.11.7 What Help / Support Do You Need to Do This?

This is a key question. Many people forget others who can help and support them to achieve behaviour change goals. This question may also draw out with whom they need to share their goals and what is needed from those people. For example, someone planning to quit smoking may need to ask smoking friends not to offer them cigarettes or not to smoke around them in the first few weeks. It may be the same for our animal owners. Thinking about the owner of Sandy the dog, it may be that she will need to talk to other family members, discuss the weight loss goals, and the plan for this. She might ask that Sandy isn't given treats or anything else outside his set mealtimes.

10.11.8 Who Else Can Help You with This Goal?

This could be family, friends, colleagues, but do guide the owner to think about animal health and welfare workers and professionals such as you too!

For some people, it may be useful to include good online communities that provide evidence-based support and mutual help. This question can also lead the owner to think about other sources of support such as groups, classes, and charities. This may be an opportunity to use the ask-offer-ask model (9.7–9.8) if there is information that they would like from you. If there is something you know about, but which the owner appears to be unaware of, make a tentative offer of this information (9.9).

10.11.9 Is There Anything Else You Need or Any Other Information to Help You?

It is very likely you know of something that the owner hasn't thought about or is not aware of. This question opens up for the owner to add anything else that they can think of, even some wild cards which can be surprising, yet often productive.

Again, ask-offer-ask (9.8) may come into play here if they ask for information from you. This can also be an opportunity to offer information (9.9) or a thought such as, 'I know of some other sources of help that possibly could be of use to you – are these something you would like to hear about or to have some information about?'

Box 10.9 Exercise

What changes / activities / tasks are you good at setting goals for / planning?
   What and how do you do this?
   Is there anything that you are not so good at setting goals for / planning?
   If so, what do you make of this?

Box 10.10 Exercise

Own goals / planning

Part 1: *Think of a goal you might like to set for yourself. It could be anything: health, work, or home related.*
   Is your goal specific? Do you need to chunk it down a bit or refine it?
   Now ask yourself these questions:

- *What might be the small first steps towards my goal?*
- *What might get in the way of me working towards or achieving this goal?*
- *How might I overcome these pitfalls?*
- *What methods have I found helpful in the past to achieve this or other goals?*
- *What is the most realistic / easily achievable of these solutions?*
- *What can I realistically do by...?*

- *What help / support do I need to do this?*
- *Who else can help me with this goal?*
- *Is there anything else I need or any other information to help me?*

Part 2: Supporting others' goals and action planning
Now find a willing friend or colleague who would be prepared to work on a goal and action plan with you and practice again – this time with their issue. It is useful if this practice person is in the preparation stage for the change that they have identified.

10.12 Contingency Plans and What May Get in the Way For People – What May Cause Trip Ups or Slip Ups?

10.12.1 Time Trips and Slips

Time trips and slips can be because there is insufficient time to do the required changes, or can be either the goal and action plan not being timely or being affected by specific time-related events.

One of the most common complaints for anyone when trying to make changes is that we struggle to find the time needed. When my colleagues and I are teaching behaviour change to both human health and animal health and welfare workers, the biggest concern we hear from workers about using the ideas we teach and described in this book is...

> '*I don't have time to do these extra things.*'

Think about your responses as you worked through this book, even just this chapter about goal setting, action, and contingency planning. You have very probably thought – this is a whole load of work I don't have time for! Which would be a completely understandable response.

When we feel we don't have time, or something will take too long, we shift back to old behaviours. Similarly, when trying new or amended ways of working with people, we can revert to those traditional methods of telling people, which don't work, or don't work consistently and in the long term (Chapter 2).

Just like the difficulties we may have in changing the way we work, so it is for our owners and the changes they want, or need to make. Time is often the biggest obstacle in all of our minds when considering change. Change is hard. It is easier in the short term to stay the same; it takes less effort. But in the long term, staying the same doesn't work or it causes more problems and inevitably more work. So it is for us with owners. A little time now supporting people to goal set, make action plans and a contingency plan is likely to have better outcomes down the road for all involved. Time well spent now also reduces the likelihood of more time spent dealing with the issue repeatedly in the future.

When people identify time as a big obstacle to change we can help by working to evoke change talk (4.10.2) from them. We can support them to remember why the change is important and to help improve their confidence to make the change (7.10). It may be useful to return to the importance, confidence and readiness scales (7.11). A return to exploring ambivalence (8.3) may also be helpful, or the hypothetical look over the fence (9.3), as well as perhaps a timeline (7.3). Using these structures can help the individual identify other things needed, perhaps more preparation before change is attempted. A word of warning: continue to watch out for that fixing reflex (2.2.8) that afflicts us as workers. We can get ahead of the owner due to a desire for change to happen (premature focus 4.6), undoing the good work thus far achieved. If a mindful and neutral (4.10.4) approach is not maintained, we can become unhelpful to an owner, and all that good work can slip through our fingers.

I often think that helping someone at the preparation stage is not unlike decorating a room in our home. It is often said that a good decorating job is all about the preparation, which takes time with the rubbing down, preparing, filling. To get a behaviour change to stick and be successful over the long term, preparation is key.

When an owner is thinking about a contingency plan, they may identify events or specific times that could impede making or consolidating the change. All of us can probably relate to specific times of the year that will hinder any good intentions of eating healthily, not drinking too much, or ensuring adequate exercise and sleep. Christmas and other festivals are very often times that trip us all up, even for a few days or perhaps weeks. Big events in our lives such as weddings can hinder behaviour changes (3.4).

For example, Sandy's owner may do really well with the goal, the action plan, and the contingency plan until they get to Christmas or go on a family holiday.

10.12.2 Physical Trip and Slips

Owners may do well with their change by using an action plan, until a physical problem occurs. This could be as simple as a common cold or a more serious virus. Something that lays them low for a few days causing a loss of rhythm of routine, motivation, or the ability to continue the change. A more serious or long-term physical issue can create significant disruption.

Often, this slip can be viewed as a failure. It can generate thoughts such as there is no point restarting the changed behaviour, and as a result there is a return to old, unwanted ways of behaving.

For owners, especially those with animals that need exercising, such as dogs or large animals, a physical issue can present significant barriers to starting or continuing a change. Physical pain is something we can all recognise as having an impact on activity and energy. Sleep deprivation is another physical issue that can make change hard to start or sustain.

10.12.3   Emotional Trips and Slips

Unexpected or emotionally laden events such as bereavements and funerals can trip people up, as can other home, emotional, life, and work issues. Other emotionally charged events that bring happiness can also have an impact – think of weddings and holidays or family celebrations and get-togethers with friends.

10.12.4   Cognitive or Thinking Trips and Slips

How a person thinks about themselves can have a huge impact on whether change can be made and sustained. Someone who has, for example, been made redundant from their job, or furloughed, may find that this affects how they view themselves and their abilities and can easily have a knock-on effect on any behaviour change.

10.12.5   Situational Trips and Slips

Finding oneself in a situation that is associated with, or linked to, an old behaviour can cause a slip up. For example, many of those who stop smoking have found a particular place or group of people a trigger to 'just have the one' cigarette again.

Often, these situational cues can be powerful because they have not yet or have rarely been experienced since the change was started. One of my colleagues stopped smoking many years ago and after the first couple of weeks, the nicotine cravings abated. They no longer thought about it much at certain points on their commute where a cigarette would have been routinely lit in the past. The repeated exposure meant that they managed the initial cravings, and it quickly became normal on the commute not to smoke. However, then they were going on holiday, an activity which they did far less frequently than their commute. Upon arrival at the airport where, in the past they would have smoked a number of cigarettes outside before checking in, they suddenly had huge cravings.

Although I stopped smoking over two decades ago, I still get a craving when I put up and decorate my Christmas tree. It is now the only time I get the urge to smoke. This may sound odd at first, but consider how many times I have been exposed to this prompt to smoke: just over 20 times.

Therefore, it can be useful to ask owners to think about events or situations that occur infrequently but could be problematic. These can then be planned for and added to the contingency plans. By helping people do this, we can assist them to have the best chance of being successful with a behaviour change.

10.12.6 Interpersonal Trips and Slips

Interpersonal issues that can trip people up might be less easy to identify or may be more subtle. Tensions or difficulties between family members or in households may cause problems in undertaking and maintaining a behaviour change. Others who may be close to the animal or animals, or to the owner, may lack understanding about the reasons or need for change. This can range from mere inconsistencies within the household in managing the animal to outright sabotage and opposition to required changes.

For example, with equine owners this can easily happen on DIY, part DIY, or full livery yards. Other horse owners, the yard owner, or yard workers can undo changes that the owner makes. When you are just one person up against the differing opinions of others, it can be hard not to succumb to the group thinking or pressure. This is not uncommon for issues such as overfeeding, access to grass, the weight or condition of animals, and even euthanasia. Equine welfare colleagues report that owners often experience pressure from others who question decisions they have made around euthanasia. Euthanasia and the decisions involved can be some of the most difficult to make in animal ownership, but when others criticise or oppose these, it can be very hard indeed, both emotionally and practically.

10.13 A Model to Help in Problem-Solving – Falloon's Model

Many animal health and welfare workers have abundant problem-solving skills. Not every owner has these abilities, or those that do have abilities might not apply them to their animals. Therefore, people may need a little support or prompting to solve problems.

The problem-solving model, by Falloon et al. (2007), might for some people be useful to generate ideas and plans in a structured way. It can be used with just one individual or can be undertaken with a group of people, for example, a couple or a family who need to work together to make behaviour changes for their animal or animals. It encourages people to collaborate to find a solution and can reduce difficulties within groups. It has six steps and is very simple. This process tends to work best when ideas are quickly jotted down.

See below for details about how to use Fallon's problem-solving model.

Box 10.11   Falloon's Model

Step 1: Identify exactly what the problem is.
Step 2: List all possible solutions.
Step 3: Highlight main advantages and disadvantages.
Step 4: Choose the 'best' solution.
Step 5: Plan exactly how to carry out the solution. Date and time review.
Step 6: Review progress.

Step 1: Identify exactly what the problem is
Similar to identifying agendas, the problem to be worked on needs to be clear and specific, not broad or hazy. Focus on one problem at a time. The owner or owners may need to be guided by the worker to break down the issues into specific problems and then identify which one to work through the process with first.

Step 2: List All Possible Solutions
Ask the owner/s to list all possible solutions they can think of. If there is more than one person, ensure everyone adds ideas, including children if they are present. Kids have great ideas that are simple, creative, and often really useful.

Note down all the solutions generated, encourage all thoughts and ideas, no matter how ridiculous or outlandish. Thank each person for their ideas. Just get the list down and don't seek comments from people, or comment yourself. If people want to discuss any possible solutions and the strengths or weaknesses of these, ask them to hold the thought and remind them that this can be done in the next stage.

When five or six solutions have been generated, move to the next step.

Step 3: Highlight the Main Advantages and Disadvantages
Now people can discuss their reactions and thoughts to each solution. Take each solution in turn and identify at least one advantage and one disadvantage for each solution but keep the discussion brief and factual. If the owner, or owners, start to generate plans here, say that this will be done in the next stage. Ensure everyone is heard and that no one person dominates.

Step 4: Choose the 'Best' Solution
In this step, a discussion can be had about the advantages and disadvantages of each listed solution. Active listening and summarising from the worker is crucial in this stage. Now, the optimal solution can be chosen. If there is more than one person involved in the discussion and two different solutions are strongly favoured by individuals, seek a compromise by asking them to agree which solution to try first and which second.

You can now remind and clarify with the person or the group the chosen solution that they will work on.

Step 5: Plan Exactly How to Carry Out the Solution. Date and Time Review
Here, you might support the owner or owners by using the goal planning template (10.9) already given. Identify obstacles or slips and trips that might get in the way of achieving the solution and add this to the contingency plan.

Step 6: Review Progress
All plans need to be reviewed regularly, and with this problem solving model it is no different.

10.14 Regularly Reviewing Goals

Goals need to be regularly reviewed, especially in the early stages of a behaviour change. People will need support to keep going and workers have an important role to play here. We consider this in more detail in next chapter, especially at 11.4 and 11.8.

10.15 Support to Build Confidence and Self-efficacy

Keeping the status quo or putting off change for another day, week or year can be appealing when we start to consider a change, when we feel how hard it is, and realise how much energy it will take. Perhaps, if a person has failed at previous change attempts (and who hasn't!), it can sap their strength, self-esteem (11.14), self-efficacy (11.15) and confidence. For some, it may feel impossible to change due to a lack of self-efficacy or if they have a belief that change is not possible for them.

Therefore, when people prepare for change and a move into action and draw up goals and action plans, they may need help to build confidence to make the change and to develop or even discover self-efficacy. Much more about how this can be done can be found in the next chapter, particularly at 11.6 and 11.12 to 11.16.4.

10.16 Goals for Welfare Issues

It is worth mentioning that in some cases, especially in welfare cases, it is not always appropriate for the goals to be entirely the owner's. It may well be that workers will need to take time to find and negotiate shared goals, when they have a different viewpoint than the owner's. Obviously, this is not easy, but it is not impossible and all of the skills and techniques we have discussed in previous chapters will support this. Being transparent about what needs to happen for the animal or animals, balanced with a neutrality (4.10.4), curiosity, and a desire to understand the other person's side of the issue, takes effort and skill from the worker. But if good engagement and rapport (6.5) has been built, combined with the owner feeling that they have personal choice and responsibility (4.10.4), then it is very possible.

10.17 Conclusion

In this chapter, thinking about preparation for action, we have at last arrived at goals. In addition, the importance of action planning (or the filling that makes it a sandwich rather than just basic and boring pieces of bread) has been explored.

We are moving through the stages of change and have covered most of the ideas, structures, skills, and techniques, apart from the essential maintenance stage and building self-efficacy which are covered in the next chapter. As this chapter has covered the preparation stage, this summary includes an exercise, detailed below, as preparation for the final elements of the book.

This is an invitation for you to consider what an action plan might look like, if you decide to use ideas and information in this book. You are invited, if it is right for you, to consider making a behaviour change: to adapt how you work with owners and others. How much you use the ideas in this book will be your decision, your personal choice and responsibility. You may choose to adopt some elements but not others, building on or touching up the ways you already work. Or you may think about overhauling or making some significant changes to how you have conversations with some owners.

Box 10.12   Exercise

Goal (*suggested*)	Action plan	Timescales	Who can help?
Using MI and other supporting ideas in my practice with animal owners, and others, to help them think about / make changes (this is a suggestion only, please amend to make it your goal).			

Now ask yourself these questions:

What might be the small first steps towards this goal?
What might get in the way of working towards or achieving this goal?
How do I think I can overcome these pitfalls?
What methods have I found helpful in the past to achieve this or other goals?
What is the most realistic / easily achievable of these solutions?
What do I think I can realistically do by...?
What help / support do I need to do this?
Who else can help me with this goal?
Is there anything else I need or any other information to help me?
What techniques / skills / ideas from the book have I thought about or used so far?
How did they go? What does this tell me about what I might need to do...?

You might now think about what might trip you up, when you might slip back to more traditional methods of working with owners. Perhaps use the contingency plan below for this.

Goal	What might get in the way of your goal and action plan?	When? How?	Contingency plan

---

Reference

Falloon, I., Barbieri, L. Boggian, I. et al. (2007). Problem solving training for schizophrenia: Rationale and review. *Journal of Mental Health* 16 (5): 553–568, DOI: 10.1080/09638230701494910.

11

Supporting People to Move into Action

11.1   Introduction

This chapter is about what we have been waiting for – action!

The previous chapter looked at goal-setting, action planning, and contingency planning and how individual, personalised, and detailed plans are important. Once we have helped someone to set goals and develop plans, how can we support them to make that leap into action?

It may appear that the action stage has been a long time coming in this book. After all, the reason you are reading it is because you want things to change, to be different for people and their animals. You probably want action and change. However, laying the groundwork, the preparation for change, is essential. If this is not done, change rarely happens successfully in ways that will stick and last.

As mentioned in Chapter 10, if you have ever done home decoration, you may be familiar with the saying 'it is all in the preparation'. Behaviour change is similar. Decorating requires all the cleaning, the rubbing down, and filling of walls and woodwork. Furniture and other items need clearing out and moving. Then, there are the difficult choices about materials and paints to use, colours, and types. It can be a real faff. But, if preparation is done well, which can seem such hard work and take time, there comes the point when the decorating suddenly seems to come together: we are flying. Paint is going on and we stand back every so often and look at our hard work. Suddenly, we can see the results and it is worth it. Even though we may have some way to go to finish the job, we now have an idea of what it will look like and can feel energised and confident in achieving what we set out to do.

How can we support people to have the same type of experience, of undertaking the preparation and getting the groundwork right to support them to make behaviour changes that will benefit them, others, and especially their animals?

Practical Human Behaviour Change for the Health and Welfare of Animals,
First Edition. Bronwen Williams.
© 2024 John Wiley & Sons Ltd. Published 2024 by John Wiley & Sons Ltd.
Companion website: www.wiley.com/go/williams/human

11.2   When to Start a Behaviour Change

Katy Milkman in her book *How to Change* says that successful changes often start at points that feel like a new start or a fresh page, and when ingrained patterns or habits are less likely to kick in. This could be on a particular day of the week, a meaningful date, after a particular life event, transition or a crisis. Milkman has shown that we think about time as 'episodes' divided up by experiences, e.g. jobs, places we have lived, and so on. This thinking about time as episodes can help people to start new behaviours. If people feel that it is a new start, a clean sheet in some way, or what Milkman calls 'resets', then they are more likely to start a new behaviour – perhaps Mondays, first day of the month, New Year's day or first day of spring.

Opportunities to reset could be, for example, anniversaries or a significant event such as a wedding, divorce, or moving home. Other resets could be because of a crisis, a human or animal health event or some other defining moment. For those working in animal welfare, it could be that you have visited the owner or that there is the possibility of prosecution or animals being removed. Contact with an owner by a welfare worker could be all that is needed to provide the opportunity for a reset.

A crisis can be a watershed moment for a few people, motivating them to move into the action stage (3.6). For some workers, there is a belief that shock tactics are the way to force an owner to make changes. Shock tactics belong with those traditional methods (Chapter 2) of trying to make people change behaviours and rarely result in behaviour change or a change that is consistent and long term. Shock tactics are more likely to result in disengagement by the owner. However, workers often believe that their shock tactics have worked. What is more likely is that, at these watershed moments, the owner perceives a crisis and a turning point or a reset. It is likely such an owner has been quietly brewing in contemplation (3.4) and is ready for a change. An animal health or welfare crisis can provide that opportunity for a reset.

Change needs energy (3.4), and a health or welfare crunch time can generate that heat to get someone moving along the stages of change and shifting the balance of their ambivalence (see 4.9). Therefore, not uncommonly, this can be wrongly interpreted as shock tactics working, and workers believing that they have the power to make someone change. We know behaviour change isn't like this; the owner is the only one who can make their changes. When the shock tactics approach is applied and change happens, it is *despite* the intervention, not because of it, or it can merely be cheap change. Cheap change (3.4) is when a person makes a quick decision to make a change without sufficient or any thought or contemplation, planning and consideration. Cheap change looks like a swift resolution, but a return to the unwanted behaviour is equally as swift.

A health or welfare crisis can definitely be a time to facilitate change, sometimes significant and rapid change. The approaches and skills covered in this book, when implemented by workers in what might be a crisis for an owner, can facilitate good and lasting change.

11.3 Supporting Resets

How can we support the creation or generation of reset opportunities for animal owners? How can we harness this information about how people view time and new starts or what Milkman calls resets?

If, as part of our work, we offer people recording sheets, it can be helpful to look at when these documents indicate a start. For example, diary sheets that start on a Monday help people to start new behaviours more on Mondays. If a weekly sheet begins on a Sunday, then starting on a Sunday is more likely. Knowing this is useful. We might use blank weekday sheets and when seeing clients or owners, perhaps put the next day as the first day on the sheet: for example a Wednesday. Then ask them to return to see us, or for us to follow up on the same day the following week or a few weeks hence. Chapter 14 includes some recording templates that may be useful.

Another way to support people to think about new starts and clean slates, is to ask and listen for what may help the person think about time episodes and resets. Ask about, or notice on the computer records if the animal's birthday is imminent, when the animal was first registered with your practice or came to the owners. Perhaps, the seasons are important to them, and if that is the case, explore how this may be helpful or what the start of a new month may mean to them.

I have come across colleagues who are into astrology, not something evidence-based perhaps, but I have been struck by some who will spend time setting intentions each new moon. They allow themselves extra opportunities for resets due to their beliefs. How can we tap into our clients, and owners' beliefs and frames of reference (Chapter 1) to look for opportunities to support them in making starts and moving into the action stage of change?

11.4 Supporting People When They Are Starting to Make Change and Moving into Action

As workers, there can be the temptation to think our job is done when people move into the action phase of change and begin to work towards their goals and desired outcomes (Chapter 10). Support from professionals, services, organisations, formal and informal, friends and family often ends at this point. We can say, 'Well done! Keep it up!' and leave them to it. However, it is often in this stage that people need as much, if not more, support than the preceding stages of change.

Change is hard, it takes effort and energy and it can be exhausting. It is often easier to drift back to old behaviours and give up when things don't go quite right, rather than persist with a change. We can soon forget our original reasons for change and remember fondly the reasons for the old behaviour. Therefore, people need to be supported in the first tentative steps in the action stage and also when life and events can trip them up. They will need support and help to reconsider and redevelop their action plans (10.9) and contingency plans (10.10) in light of the new experiences and information garnered from making the change and associated trips and slips (10.12) along the way. Often, when people (including us) start to make a change, high energy is experienced combined with relief that we are actually undertaking change. But, as time goes on, it can be hard to remember the reasons why the change was needed, and slipping back into old behaviours, just for a day or so and then for longer, can become appealing.

Therefore, there is a continued role for workers or others in helping the individual to review their goals and progress regularly, to tweak their action plans (10.9) and to refine their contingency plans (10.10).

Box 11.1   Losing Excitement and Focus for Change

If you have ever started a diet, you perhaps were very focused at the start on all the healthy things you would eat, how good it would be for you, and other reasons for the change. You may have stocked your fridge with appropriate food items and even bought new recipe books. You may then have, like me, experienced that drift and change in thinking as the diet progressed, got a bit boring or you didn't lose as much weight as you would have liked. The thoughts of sugars, refined carbohydrates, and lovely fats, often combined into delicious baked items, start to become very attractive and enticing.

In human health behaviour change, we know that regular rewards can support behaviour changes and help people to keep going. For example, some people who stop smoking choose to put the money that they would have spent on cigarettes to one side to use for special treats.

Rewards may seem not so easy or appropriate for animal health, care, and welfare work. But it has been found that one of the best, most effective rewards when changing behaviour is simply support from another person. Someone who consistently gives unconditional (4.10.4) feedback on, and support for, both the progress and any struggles experienced. Someone who is really in the person's corner. This support from another is best in small amounts but offered frequently and regularly. We might think about a dosing approach: small doses but administered sufficiently often or regular brief interventions to maintain progress.

Box 11.2   Quick Exercise

Think about your role and what methods may be available to you to offer regular brief support to people making a change and in the maintenance stage.
It may not need to be a consultation or a visit. What other ways may be possible?
Use of technology comes in useful here: texts, emails, and other methods.
What might work for you, your role and your clients or owners?

11.5   People Need Practical Skills to Make Changes or Do What We Ask, Advise or Prescribe

It is easy to assume that people have the skills, ability, confidence, or knowledge to undertake what is asked of them for the health, care, or welfare or their animals. This may well not be the case. Rather, we may need to demonstrate, explain, or model what is required.

As a mental health nurse most of my work was in the community, and therefore I am very used to giving depot intramuscular injections to adults in large muscles. When I became a vaccinator during the Covid-19 pandemic, I initially struggled with giving smaller injections into a different and smaller muscle: the deltoid. My colleagues assumed that, as I was a nurse, I would be fine with a different injection site! When my elderly cat needed subcutaneous injections each month, my vet and friend assumed I would competent and confident to administer them. I found many an excuse to get her to do his injections, including invites of lunch or tea and cake and then mentioning that his injection was due and might she like to do it. My experience and confidence were lacking for what my friend would see as a very simple injection.

Physical ability may be another issue that can be missed. Animal medication is often fiddly, comes in foil wrappers, in screw top bottles, and small syringes. These may take some skill and reasonable eyesight to use. Some owners may have difficulties with grip or dexterity in their hands or have poor eyesight and struggle to use what is routinely given out.

Others can have literacy problems, dyslexia, or have a different first language. Some with learning difficulties or cognitive issues such as dementia may need clearer and simpler instructions, and pictures or symbols can be of help here.

Box 11.3   Example

One of my veterinary nursing friends told me about a client who gave her companion animal a topical flea treatment orally. The nurse wondered how on earth this could have happened. We talked about how some people have poor or no literacy and are too ashamed to admit it. Those with dyslexia may struggle with the detailed information that comes with medication. Perhaps that owner may only have experienced medication given orally, or their experience may have previously been with humans and not animals. As we talked about this case, this veterinary nurse also wondered if everyone will automatically be able to use the calibration on syringes. This demonstrates how easily we can assume people have the skills needed to undertake tasks, to care for their animals and to make required behaviour changes.

11.6   Building Confidence for Action

A lack of confidence is often the biggest issue for many people when a change is first considered. Anything that reduces confidence throughout the action (3.6), maintenance and even termination stages (3.7) will impact on the individual and their ability to make changes. The person may believe that they cannot make the change or that they will fail. Many people will have attempted changes in the past and returned to old behaviours and now view this as a failure. Perhaps most of us have had such experiences and can identify with this.

11.7   Stages of Change

The evidence indicates that people often travel through the different stages of change a number of times (3.9) before successfully changing a behaviour. Just knowing that this is normal, especially for big changes, can be helpful to people considering change but who feel disheartened and wonder if it is even worth trying to do something different. Remembering that the stages of change are cyclical can be enlightening, and showing owners The Stages of Change Model and explaining it can be really helpful.

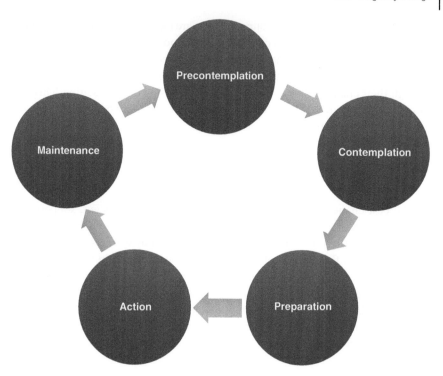

As workers we can also have our expectations of owners: that they will just get on, make the change and all will be well. When owners delay the change or revert to previous behaviours perhaps after some success, we can despair and view them as failing. Regarding people this way, when they are trying to make changes, is unfair. Workers too can be downhearted and despondent when owners cycle through the stages of change. Feeling this way doesn't help with job or role satisfaction. When an owner doesn't do what has been advised, or even what they have agreed to, workers can judge them fairly harshly. Workers may also question their own skills or the job role.

Rather than viewing a return to an old unwanted behaviour as a failure, it can be reframed (1.2) as very usual and a normal slip or trip up (10.12). In behaviour change, it is very common to have a go, hit difficulties, and return to old behaviour or undertake the new behaviour sporadically. Using the car journey analogy, we wouldn't plan for a journey and set out only to return home when a diversion or traffic queue was encountered, stating that we had failed and were never trying that journey again! We would very probably find a way around, even if we got to the destination a bit late and via an unexpected route. We may even learn something along the way, even if it is the need to check the weather forecast next time or leave more time for surprises on journeys.

If owners can understand that slips and trips are likely and that obstacles (10.12) will occur, more realistic goals can be set (10.4) and action plans devised accordingly (10.9). Robust contingency plans can be devised too (10.10) for when things go awry. We as workers, similarly, can be more forgiving and support people through their change process, rather than just focusing on goal-setting. This can enhance workers' own feelings of an ability to help owners change and improve the welfare of their animals.

11.8   Keeping on Track

For the best chance for change working and becoming consistent, support and regular reviews of goals and plans (10.14) are essential, especially at the start of the action stage (3.6). This doesn't have to be provided by workers if owners have identified within their action plans (10.9) others who will help them. It doesn't need to be face-to-face either. A quick text or email from a worker to remind an owner to keep going can work wonders or an owner may choose to report into their worker by text or email to say they are on target. These prompts or reporting in activities can be added to the action plans (10.9). I have used these methods with good success over many years with hard-to-engage clients in my mental health work.

Box 11.4   Example

In my human health work, I found that for some patients, a plan for them to just email or text me regularly between meetings worked really well. They didn't need a response from me, rather just telling me was enough, and it gave me information to start the next face-to-face meeting with them.

In the action stage (3.6), it can be helpful for people to have physical reminders, prompts, or cues. You may be able to offer diaries or recording sheets. If you don't have anything suitable available, design something simple. A checklist may be useful for some, something that they can tick off (see Chapter 14 for an example). There is good evidence that checklists work well in assisting people to ensure they complete tasks. Atul Gawande's book titled *The Checklist Manifesto* (2009) describes how the use of tick lists for completed simple tasks has massively reduced incidents and safety issues in the human health world and the aviation industry. Simple checklists work for these big safety issues, and can really help owners with their own actions.

I often suggest to equine welfare workers that they might supply an owner with a basic whiteboard on which to write down tasks to tick off when done. This simple aid can make a real difference. Most of us will be accustomed to using whiteboards to organise and plan within clinical settings. These are used in both animal and in human health care. We understand the usefulness of this, but owners may not know, or have thought, about it.

These are all ideas that may support the action stage, but don't force them on people. Many people don't tell others when they have literacy problems, so these methods might be inappropriate for some and cause them to back off from working towards change.

However, recording sheets, checklists, and diaries can be really useful for owners to bring and share with us, should they want to, at subsequent meetings, appointments, or visits. There is good evidence that when documentation is used, patterns and issues are more easily identified and recognised. Also, people can experience a feeling of mastery, or achievement (11.16.1) when they review what they have done.

Sharing these records with a worker, or someone else supportive, can be very helpful and encourage an individual to keep going with a behaviour change even when things are tough. When an owner hasn't managed to implement their action plans (10.9) consistently, this information can be useful to help to identify what tripped them up (10.12) and what can be learnt and so be added to a contingency plan (10.10). If you do use recording sheets or checklists with your owners, remember to ask about these and ensure a review of them. If an owner is asked to document and record but then not asked about it, they are likely to stop and may even disengage from working with us.

11.9   Habit Stacking / Chaining

Habit stacking or chaining is another idea that may be of use for some owners. We all habit stack: where automatic well-established habits prompt us to do another task, chore, or activity. If a new, desired activity is linked to an already established one, it can be easier to remember and to add into daily or weekly routine. A habit stack of mine was to keep my aged cat's medication on a shelf above the kettle. This meant I always remembered to give his morning medication when making my first cup of tea in the morning. This, however, wouldn't have worked for someone who was used to getting up late, rushing out of the door, and getting a coffee on the way to work. They would have needed another prompt, maybe to put the medication next to their toothbrush or something similar that would work for them.

Box 11.5   Quick Exercise

Checklists

Think about what checklists and visual reminders you use. How do these work for you? Could you use them more for you? Can you use checklists and reminders more with owners? If so, where, when and how?

Habit Stacking

Now think about very regular habits you have, those automatic without fail types of behaviours. What are they? Can you list these? Now think about some brief activities you would like to add to your day. It could be a very quick thing that you want to do but keep forgetting or don't do regularly. Maybe it is remembering people's birthdays or taking the rubbish out of your car.

It might look something like this:

When I make my first cup of tea / coffee, I will check my diary for any birthdays or anniversaries or other important events.

or

When I remove my keys out of the ignition, I will collect up any rubbish and take it with me when I leave the car.

Another useful tool is dosette medication boxes that owners can use to set up medications to be given for the week ahead. These are easily obtainable on the internet or from high street chemists and can act as a handy visual reminder of what needs to be given, and when. Just be aware if the owner has their own human medication in a dosette box too, clear labelling of the boxes will be needed. My mother didn't use dosette boxes but managed to take her Labrador's tablet one morning and give him her medication. Thankfully, neither of them came to any harm. This does demonstrate however, the need to work out appropriate, manageable and helpful methods for each individual.

Many countries have increasingly ageing populations, numbers of whom live with complex comorbidities requiring many medications. Medication for their animals can add to that burden and with potential for confusion and accidents. For some, symbols rather than words may be more helpful as reminders.

Most of us now have a number of electronic devices and gizmos, including mobile phones, computers, and smart speakers. Alarms and reminders can be set up on these which can be very helpful prompts for many people.

Box 11.6   Example
A lovely former neighbour of mine, a retired nurse, would have an alarm on her phone several times a day to remind her to give her husband, who had Parkinson's disease, his medication. This was so much part of her life that often, when we were outside talking, her phone would bleep and even I recognised it and would say to her, 'Oh, Henry's medication is due!'

11.10   Cue Card Prompts

Cue cards may be useful for an owner who has difficulties in certain situations. For some people, this could be simple helpful prompts when they are disheartened or struggling. The owner should generate the wording to ensure it is specific to them and their situation, but workers can support them to do this. It could be as simple as 'keep going' or 'it will be worth it'. A different example could be where someone with too many animals or at risk of moving into hoarding finds themselves tempted to take on more animals. Prewritten cue cards can help them move away from the urge to take on another creature. In this case, a cue card could also have phrases or examples of what the person might say to someone who is trying to offer them an animal. The cue cards prompts should be written by the individual, when they are calm and not under pressure, perhaps with your assistance

When drawing up or reviewing goals (10.4) and action plans (10.14), considering what obstacles could cause a trip or slip up (3.9, 10.12), and designing contingency plans (10.10), you could ask the individual to also think about statements that could be helpful should they lose heart, waver or not do identified actions. These can then be written up on cue cards.

Using file cards or something similar, ask the person to write down statements that would be helpful to them when things get difficult. These could be a phrase that someone they trust might say to them. It could be what you as a worker might say to help them keep going and stay on track.

It has been found that referring to yourself in the second person (i.e. **You** have the ability to do this) rather than the first person (i.e. **I** have the ability to do this) can be more helpful. Statements made in the second person seem to have more of an affect and can feel, for some, almost like someone else is physically with them and supporting them.

11.11   Examples of Potential Cue Card Statements

'You have faced difficulties before and have managed them and have even learnt from them such as when...'	'You CAN manage this...'
'It will be worth it in the end when you reach your goal of...'	'You are not responsible for all the animals in the world, and you can't be.'
	'You are not able to take on any more animals, you have rules and limits.'

11.12   Listing Achievements

When life becomes difficult or obstacles or roadblocks occur, it is common for many of us to become stuck into familiar patterns of focusing on what has not worked, has gone wrong or upon perceived failures. Listing the person's achievements over the years, no matter what these are, can be useful to revisit when this happens. A timeline (7.3) may illuminate the person's achievements and can be listed in a quick-to-read and accessible format, if that suits them. This helps a move away from focusing on what is going wrong or feels hopeless and can remind people of the bigger picture, so helping develop self-efficacy (11.15) when there are challenges.

Box 11.7   Exercise

Quickly jot down your achievements. This could be over a short period or a longer one, or perhaps even over your life.

Achievements in the past month	Achievements in the past year	Achievements in your lifetime

Now review these and consider how it feels when you reflect on them.
And now perhaps, identify any patterns or what these achievements tell you about yourself? About what has helped you succeed?
What do these say to you about the future and any changes that you might make?

11.13   Helping People Make Change – How They See Themselves in Relation to Behaviour Change

This section explores how people feel or think about themselves and about change and how we can help them to be more successful. Self-esteem is considered and then self-efficacy.

11.14   Self-esteem

Self-esteem is important for change. If self-esteem is lacking, it may be very difficult for an owner to envisage making a change. They may feel unable to make a change or even that they are not worth the effort involved. Some who lack self-esteem may even say to themselves, and others, 'What's the point? I will only screw it up.'

Workers can help a little with this. Many of the ideas already outlined in previous chapters can assist the worker and owner. Support the owner to consider the reasons for staying the same and the reasons for change by exploring ambivalence (8.3). You can develop understanding of the history of how they got to this point, by hearing, exploring and using a timeline (7.3). Hear the beliefs and concerns and the context of the issues for the owner right now. All those important skills of active listening (Chapter 5) with empathy (5.15) and without judging the individual (4.10.4) will be essential.

The core ideas, or the spirit, of motivational interviewing (4.5, 4.10) will be key. Also, go at the owner's pace whilst not being tempted to try telling, persuading, or cajoling them into making the change (those traditional methods of (not) getting people to make change in Chapter 2). Avoid generating the answers or solutions for the owner; resist the fixing reflex (2.2.8). Nothing is more damaging for someone's confidence and self-esteem than feeling useless and disenabled when someone else takes over.

11.15   Self-efficacy

Closely linked to feelings of self-esteem is self-efficacy. Some of the ideas to develop and increase self-efficacy can be helpful when supporting owners, including when they are in the preparation (3.5), action (3.6), and then maintenance (3.7) stages of change as well as the activities of action planning (10.9), reviewing plans (10.14) and contingency planning (10.10).

> Self-efficacy is the internal belief or,
> *'Confidence that a person has in their own ability to successfully influence their surroundings by completing a certain task or solving a problem'* (Bandura 1977).

Self-efficacy is important for behaviour change as an owner's belief in their ability to make change can be fundamental in whether change happens or not.

Self-efficacy is internal and personal. It could be influenced by past experiences and by an individual's frame of reference (Chapter 1). We can't give other people self-efficacy. It isn't something we can inject into someone or persuade them to have.

Supporting self-efficacy in humans is similar to how we work with animals. When building confidence in animals to do something new, frightening, or stressful, it isn't possible to 'give' an animal confidence or 'make' them less stressed. Rather, we work with the animal, assisting them, finding the right way for each individual to develop and learn. Similarly, humans who are considering or need to make behaviour changes require support to find personal individual ways to develop and build their self-efficacy.

Self-efficacy can vary over time, even from day to day, if not moment to moment. It will also differ in different situations. For example, someone who has stopped smoking may feel confident about not smoking at work but less so when socialising with others who still smoke. An animal owner may experience more self-efficacy at different times of year. For example, perhaps when the summer makes behaviour changes easier than in the winter months with conditions that cause more difficulties.

Self-efficacy can drop away over time; some owners may set out on a change with good self-efficacy, feeling that they can do what is required, only for this to diminish as the pressing and important reasons why change was needed are forgotten. This may be familiar to many of us – we start out on a change, maybe diet or exercise, and feel full of hope and excitement, but the hard slog kicks in and over time, the reasons for making the change, which were imperative or in sharp focus, become more difficult to recall.

Some owners have low self-efficacy at the start and, although they might realise a change is needed, they may not believe it is possible for them. Others may begin well but when obstacles get in the way, they become quickly disheartened and consequently give up. We all have skills within us that help us make changes, but some people have fewer abilities and skills and this will impact upon their self-efficacy. For some, life circumstances at particular times may reduce their self-efficacy. So, how can we help?

Bandura identified four influencing factors for improving self-efficacy. These are outlined next with some ideas about how these four factors can be used with animal owners to help them make changes.

11.16 Four Elements for Improving Self-efficacy

Mastery experiences – Experiences gained when people take on a new challenge and succeed and which promote a sense of achievement	**Vicarious experiences** Learning by modelling on others, experiencing and seeing what others do and achieve
Verbal support The way others talk to the person about the change, the words they use, their attitudes and tone	**Emotional and physiological states** The context for the person at the time, how able they are within themselves to think about making a change

---

Box 11.8   Example

I was on a walk one day and came across a very quiet road where a father was supporting his little girl to ride her bicycle without stabilisers. This little girl was pedaling furiously, focusing on staying upright while her dad videoed this on his phone and called out words of encouragement. She was certainly having a 'mastery' experience (11.16.1), having a go and being successful. She was receiving support from her father, who was filming but most importantly giving 'verbal support' (11.16.3). I am guessing she wanted to ride a bike due to 'vicarious experiences' (11.16.2) as she probably had seen others ride a bike, perhaps her friends, older siblings, or her parents. Finally, she was very likely in a good place both physically and emotionally (11.16.4) to attempt it. If physically unwell or emotionally upset, angry, or distracted, she would not have been able to give the total and absolute concentration that she demonstrated for the task.

Riding her bike unassisted that day was building that little girl's self-efficacy, her belief that she *could* learn, do new things and be successful.

11.16.1   Improving Self-efficacy – Mastery Experiences: Gaining a Sense of Achievement

Mastery is experienced when we attempt something and gain a sense of achieving. Conscious practice of actions can be helpful to support the chance of success and reduce the likelihood of failure and so aid mastery.

There are activities for which there is little or no room for failure, such as heart surgery or flying a plane. For these, instruction, coaching, and simulated practice will be paramount in enabling the surgeon or the pilot to eventually undertake the required task with confidence in their ability. Practice reduces the chance of failure, enables quick responses and the ability to manage obstacles and challenges that will inevitably crop up, including those that are unforeseen.

Just like surgeons or pilots, owners need skills to succeed in taking on tasks or activities, including those required for behaviour changes. The best way to learn a skill or improve performance is through practice of existing skills or acquiring new ones. For behaviour changes people may need to learn new skills, build on existing ones or even reawaken or revisit dormant skills that have been unused for a while.

Once a worker has learnt about an owner and their experiences, they can then help the individual to think about what skills they need to make required behaviour changes. Again, the timeline (7.3) can be helpful here. By talking through a new timeline or revisiting a previous one, the owner can identify what skills they have successfully used in the past and what might be needed now. A look-over-the-fence or the hypothetical question (9.3) to envisage change can generate some thoughts about what skills might be needed. Exploring a typical day (7.6) may also help some owners to identify what is needed in their everyday life to enable them to succeed in making change. For some, being asked about what other people might do, those 'vicarious experiences' covered more in the next section, may help them to identify skills that they require.

We need to help the individual make a start, begin to make the change, gain momentum, and so develop a feeling that they can do it, that change is possible. Getting on and doing is essential for altering behaviours; talking about and thinking about change is important but too much can lead people to get stuck in chronic contemplation (3.4). Good, achievable and realistic goal-setting (10.4), including breaking the goals down into smaller goals and components (10.6) allows achievements to be more easily recognisable for the owner, which then supports self-efficacy. Action planning (10.9), how an owner will work towards the changes, will also be key to helping them to succeed and develop a sense of mastery, or achievement.

Contingency plans (10.10) can also help support self-efficacy. Being psychologically prepared for obstacles, trips and slips (10.12) along the way makes these easier to deal with when they occur and allows the owner to keep in sight the bigger picture and retain a focus on where they want to be. If people can recognise an obstacle, deal with it, and also gain recognition from others for overcoming it, this greatly supports self-efficacy. Owners can become more confident in making the change, to cope with and manage issues and events that get in the way. This can help owners reframe (1.2) the journey of behaviour change; recognising that not everything will go smoothly or always to plan, but they can be well prepared and able to deal with difficulties. When this happens, rather than feeling like a failure and that there is little point in continuing, owners are more likely to see themselves as successful.

It can be useful to explore where or when an owner's self-efficacy is high and where it may be less or lacking. For example, the owner of Sandy the dog may be much more confident about not feeding treats and titbits on workdays when there is structure and the rest of the family are mostly out of the house. Sandy's owner might identify her self-efficacy to be less good at weekends, evenings, or holidays such as Christmas.

Workers can help owners to gain a sense of mastery or achievement in other ways, such as asking if recording or documenting may help. For some, having written schedules or diaries can be beneficial, as can lists. Smart phones with their advanced technology offer access to apps that can record information.

Documenting each achievement, completed elements of an action plan (10.9) or keeping a diary can be a really helpful way for owners to track and observe progress and so persevere when change seems hard. Much of the behaviour change evidence suggests that documenting behaviour can be a key element for success, as what is recorded is seen. It can enable owners to identify that they may be doing better than they realise, as many of us will focus on what has not gone right rather than what has gone well and has been achieved. Documenting or recording allows people to see a more accurate picture: after all, that is one of the reasons clinicians and other workers write and keep notes or records! See Chapter 11 for a sample task and activity recording sheet.

If an owner wants to record or document, invite them to share it, if they are willing, in future appointments or visits. Being encouraged to talk through progress and experiences can support an objective view of change by the owner, as well as allowing them to gain support and recognition from another person. These records can promote a feeling of a bridge or connection between appointments with you or other workers.

A word of caution: recording is not for everyone, and therefore should not be forced upon people. If pushed when unwanted or unhelpful people can feel undermined or overwhelmed and so reduce their feelings of self-efficacy. When used inappropriately by workers, being asked to record may generate discord (4.6) and even cause owners to back away from making a change or disengage from the worker. Literacy issues may also be a reason for an owner to show hesitancy in using recording.

11.16.2 Improving Self-efficacy – Vicarious Experiences

Vicarious experiences occur when an owner sees other people doing activities or making changes. This can impact upon the owner's self-efficacy, by introducing a belief that they too might make a change. Curiously there is evidence that in friendship groups a number of life experiences often occur at the same time for people, such as engagements, marriage, pregnancies, moving house, and divorce. This may be due to similar ages in some groups, but it is also recognised that the impact of seeing friends undertaking activities and experiencing life events influences other group members' behaviour and so they are more likely to do what they see others undertake or achieve.

Therefore, one of the ways for some owners to improve self-efficacy is by witnessing others' behaviour. So, how might we help here? There are a number of ways workers can support owners to have vicarious experiences.

We might ask an owner to talk about friends, family, associates, other animal owners they know who are successful with the management of animals or for particular behaviours that the owner has identified that they too need to do, or consider doing. This may be difficult if the owner is part of a group that is hard to reach or to engage. Strong influences by family or other important people hugely affect owners. Customs and practices can be very difficult to break away from, especially if they are important in an individual's frame of reference (Chapter 1). Look for those whose behaviour demonstrates what is needed so that others can be signposted to them.

To bolster vicarious experiences, an owner might attend groups or courses if this is achievable or appropriate for them. Workers might provide information here, but remember to offer it and perhaps use the format of ask-offer-ask (9.8).

In human behaviour change, addiction support groups such as Alcoholics Anonymous, Narcotics Anonymous, and Gamblers Anonymous have helped many, many people over decades. Such groups enable those with significant difficulties to come into contact with others who have successfully made change and are in recovery. These create vicarious experiences by allowing those joining a group to realise that change is possible. Not everyone is suited to these types of groups and programmes. Similarly, for those who need to change behaviours for the welfare of their animals, groups or courses may not be for them: a one size fits all approach is to be avoided.

Another option to develop vicarious experiences are good online resources. There may be useful social media groups that can help the individual see others doing things differently or upon whom they can model their own behaviours. YouTube may be of help, as might TED Talks and other video or audio resources. There is a lot of accurate, helpful material out there, but also much that is not evidence-based or appropriate. Workers should have an idea where to direct owners for useful resources, while remembering ask-offer-ask (9.8).

Finally, don't forget that we, as workers, need to model self-efficacy. This doesn't mean that we should be absolutely perfect at everything! In fact, if we appear too capable, it can deskill or demotivate people. What we can do is to role model being confident in making changes, being tolerant of our mistakes, to persevere and not berate ourselves whilst acknowledging errors and learning from them. The language that owners hear, or overhear workers use when talking about themselves, can have an enormous impact.

11.16.3 Improving Self-efficacy – Verbal Support

The third element that can help people develop self-efficacy is verbal support from others. Interestingly, this doesn't have to be complicated or lengthy. Prochaska and DiClemente (1994) found that those successful in making and maintaining changes often received small but frequent and regular encouragement from someone else. This could make all the difference.

As will be explored in the next chapter about the maintenance stage, people often receive a lot of verbal and other support at the start, as they begin to prepare for change or early in the action stage, but this can soon wear off. As change continues and the inevitable obstacles or slips occur, owners will need help from others to stay on track and to persist.

For an owner in the preparation stage (3.5) and considering an action plan (10.9) it is worth asking who might provide them with verbal support. It may be a friend or family member, perhaps you or another professional. It could be online support that the owner can tap into.

As a worker you may feel, when reading this, that this requires a whole lot of work for which you don't have time. However, this regular support doesn't have to come from you. Support can be given by someone else in your practice or organisation – it can be just a quick but regular text message or short email. Some owners may just need someone to report to, and not need a reply, or not every time. The act of checking in can produce a feeling of support from another. We just need to remember to discuss what an owner has sent us at the next appointment with them.

If this still sounds like too much time and effort, perhaps weigh it against continuing to see the owner and their animal when there is no behaviour change. Consider how much time that scenario will take up, over the weeks, months, or even years to come, and the consequences for owners, animals, and workers, organisations and other agencies.

Finally, it may be helpful for the individual to generate their own reminders and support for themselves. If they are someone who runs an unhelpful inner dialogue such as 'I never manage things!' or 'I always screw up in the end', they may benefit from using cue cards (11.10) or even something on their phone that may help counter these thoughts. These will need to be tailored and individual but might be something like, 'Keep going, you can do this'. Or 'Small steps make big changes' or 'Just because things haven't worked out perfectly today, it doesn't ruin the goal'.

11.16.4 Improving Self-efficacy – Emotional and Physiological States

How someone is feeling emotionally and physically will affect or impact their self-efficacy. How able they are to think about, undertake, or continue to make a change can be hindered by feeling unwell, stressed, worried, or by being just generally under the weather.

While we, as workers, probably can do little to help if our client or owner is physically unwell or in pain, many of the elements discussed above can help if someone is struggling emotionally. Sometimes, supporting someone to find practical help and support for a problem can enable them to make, or maintain, a change.

Throughout this book, the importance of good quality listening has been consistently highlighted. Don't underestimate the power of this. If listening is all we can do for some people, it can be significantly helpful when offered with skill and care. At the very least, this may mean that the person can resume behaviour changes when things improve a little and that they will return to us, continue engagement and contact, and possible change is not lost.

That said, sometimes people can make swift and decisive changes when in some sort of crisis (3.4) – it can throw a spotlight on what they have been putting off. Difficulties and life events, although exhausting, can also, for some, bring a sense of energy from a crisis and a reprioritising.

Box 11.9   Exercise

Think about one or two changes you have made at any time in your life. Then, think about the four elements of self-efficacy and if any or even all applied to your change and what these were.

The change was..

What helped to make this change? Use the boxes below and then consider what this might illustrate for you.

Mastery / sense of achievement

●

●

Verbal support

●

●

Vicarious experiences

●

●

How you were physically and emotionally

●

●

Box 11.10   Exercise

If you have an opportunity, find a friend or colleague to undertake a time-line with.

Identify a behaviour that they have changed in the past, even if they have stopped, or stopped and started a number of times. As you guide them through the timeline, listen out for the four self-efficacy elements.

You can even try this yourself; however, having someone to facilitate this is usu-ally better. If you do try this, see what comes to light about your own self-efficacy, what helps to improve it, and look for times when it has been different and why this might have been.

Box 11.11   Exercise – Self-Efficacy

There are a number of simple self-efficacy tests we can do for ourselves. One, the Generalized Self-Efficacy Scale by Schwarzer and Jerusalem (1995), is quick, easy to use, and well-recognised. You can find it in the templates and appendices chapter (Chapter 14). This can bring an insight into your own, and others, self-efficacy.

Part 1

If you choose to do the self-efficacy test for yourself, work through the 10 Generalized Self-Efficacy Scale questions, and for each, mark if it is not at all true (1 point), hardly true (2 points), moderately true (3 points), or exactly true (4 points). Then add up your total points which will be somewhere between 10 and 40. A higher score indicates more self-efficacy.

Part 2

Think about a time when things were much different for you than they are now. How might your test and scores have looked then? The same? Different? If different, how and why? How would your self-efficacy then impact on how you made changes or took decisions at that time?

Part 3

Now think about someone you know, if possible, a client, owner, or perhaps a junior colleague or student who is working with you. Perhaps someone who is struggling with looking after their animal or animals or has had to make some big life decisions or could make changes in their life but doesn't. Use your imagination, and with what you know about the person, have a go at guessing what they might score on self-efficacy scale and their overall score. How might their scores look? What do you make of this?

11.17   Conclusion

This chapter has explored ways in which people can be supported to be successful in making changes, especially in the action stage. Much of the information and the ideas here come from a variety of resources, most of which are not MI. However, many if not all the ideas and structures of MI can be used to underpin and support the strategies and methods in this chapter. Crucially, the spirit of the approach and underpinning philosophy of MI (4.5) can be used throughout.

The next chapter looks at the final stage of change, maintenance, and how owners and others can continue to sustain changes they have made.

References

Bandura, A. (1977). Self-efficacy: Toward a unifying theory of behavioural change. *Psychological Review* 84 (2): 191–215. https://doi.org/10.1037/0033-295X.84.2.191

Gawande, A. (2009) *The Checklist Manifesto*. New York: Metropolitan Books.

Milkman, K. (2021) How to Change. *The science of getting from where you are to where you want to be.* London: Vermilion.

Prochaska, J., Norcross, J. and DiClemente, C. (1994) *Changing for Good*. New York: Harper Collins.

Schwarzer, R., and Jerusalem, M. (1995). Generalized self-efficacy scale. In: *Measures in Health Psychology: A User's Portfolio. Causal and Control Beliefs* (ed. J. Weinman, S. Wright, and M. Johnston), 35–37. Windsor, UK: NFER-NELSON.

12

Maintenance of Change and Beyond

12.1   Introduction

The maintenance stage (3.7), in the stages of change (Chapter 3), is often neglected by those helping people to make changes. Although by the maintenance stage the change may appear to be well embedded, there is a risk of the owner sliding back into old behaviours especially as support and interest from others falls away. This chapter looks at how to support animal owners and others when they have successfully made a behaviour change and now have to keep it going.

12.2   Maintenance Stage of Change

Maintenance was, initially, the final element of Prochaska and DiClemente's stages of change theory. Later, they would add another final stage, rather disconcertingly called the 'termination stage'. This termination stage, Prochaska and DiClemente said, is where some people can move to when they no longer have a desire to return to a previous behaviour and relapse is unlikely. In the termination stage, it can be hard for the individual to even recognise themselves as the person who did the old behaviour as it seems so foreign to who they are now. In the maintenance stage, people may still need some support, often brief, and not necessarily from workers or other professionals. In the termination stage it is not impossible for someone to slip back, but it is far less likely.

In the maintenance stage the new behaviour is embedded and becomes more routine or habitual. The previous stage, action (3.6), requires conscious thought and activity, whereas in the maintenance stage, the behaviour becomes more ingrained, and may, if we are lucky, take less effort or thought. Much is talked

Practical Human Behaviour Change for the Health and Welfare of Animals,
First Edition. Bronwen Williams.
© 2024 John Wiley & Sons Ltd. Published 2024 by John Wiley & Sons Ltd.
Companion website: www.wiley.com/go/williams/human

about timescales for change to occur or for new habits to be formed and to stick. People are always keen to know by *when* things will happen, *when* changes will be complete and behaviours no longer be a problem. There is little or no evidence for some of the timeframes in common usage, including the often cited 21 days to change a habit.

A clue for the time it takes to move from the action stage to maintenance is given by Prochaska and Prochaska (2016) who state that people who altered behaviour found it much easier to sustain those changes six to nine months on. When in the maintenance stage, people were much less likely to slip or trip up (10.12) and go back to the old behaviour. They estimated that the maintenance stage lasts for around five years, after which it is possible for some people, although by no means for all, to move into the termination stage. These, of course, are for big changes such as smoking or substance misuse.

Some of the changes we need people to make for the well-being of animals may only require adjustments or slight changes to how they do things. If a change or alteration in how an owner behaves results in life being easier, this can increase their confidence. They may have a sense of achievement (11.16.1) from making the change and from being supported in doing so. If their actions can be linked or stacked on to other habits (11.9), changes may be quick and sustained.

However, for some, significant changes need to be made to improve the welfare and care of their animals. The journey of change for these people may be comparable to those who make significant human health changes such as in an addiction. Therefore, this acts as a reminder of the importance of factoring in support for an owner over a good length of time: months, and even years for some. This support does not have to be from you. Action plans (10.9) and contingency plans (10.10) should include a variety of help and support that the individual can access and that they identify as appropriate for them.

Box 12.1   Exercise

Think about a change or changes you have made in the past. What helped you to succeed? How long did it take? What alterations did you need to make along the way? What helped? Who helped? What skills did you have that helped you change? What habits did you already have that changes were stacked upon?

Box 12.2   Time

Time, or rather the lack of it, has been discussed elsewhere in this book (11.16.3) but it is worth mentioning it again. Many readers' hearts may sink when considering the suggested change timeframes in the previous paragraph. There may be the thought, 'this is all well and good, but we don't have *time* for all of this!'

However, consider the following:

- The methods outlined in this book, when used with skill, take little or no longer than the traditional approaches.
- The strategies described do not have to be used in a linear order, rather, with practice, they become part of our conversations. While we actively listen and support change talk in owners, we can pick and choose elements or strategies to use in that moment for that person to help them.
- A little time spent at the start of the working relationship, or an episode for a particular health or welfare problem, reduces time spent down the line. We can 'frontload' and successfully invest for the future.
- These methods improve engagement resulting in fewer wasted appointments or visits.
- They reduce client or owner dissatisfaction and can help diffuse anger, hostility, and aggression.
- Using these methods reduces the likelihood of complaints, and when they do happen, they are often easier to resolve.
- For those involved in welfare, there will be cases that continue over months, years, and even decades. Sometimes they involve multiple family members and across subsequent generations. If we can reduce these by even a small number, then that can be a huge gain time-wise, as well as resource-wise.
- These methods can be used with welfare reporters, a few of whom can take up significant time for organisations and charities.
- This way of working gives workers increased job satisfaction and reduces pressure, stress, and anxiety.

Remember, that the Stages of Change Model is not a linear one, where one step is completed and then we move on to the next. As with all of human life and experience, change can be complex and there can be fluctuations. Someone can move backwards and forward through the stages of change, and this is perfectly normal. Often we will hear an owner move back and forth through several of the stages of change within a few minutes or even a few sentences. Someone might say in one breath that they need to make the change and that it is important (change talk 4.10.2). Then, in the next breath say they can't make the change right now, citing difficulties and the cost of change (sustain talk 4.9). Then, they might state that the change could be possible and even suggest time scales (preparation 3.5), then express how fearful they are of failing and wonder whether it is worth the effort (contemplation 3.4).

However, when people settle into the maintenance stage (3.7) they can appear focused, stable and that all is well, but there are still things that can trip them up. It is easy for workers, owners and others around them to become less watchful, more complacent or overly confident and to think that old behaviours are no longer a risk.

The termination stage, added at a later date by Prochaska and DiClemente, is when the change is now so integrated into day-to-day life that it can be difficult to remember what it was like before the change. A similar experience might be when we introduce an animal into our lives. After a while, they become so in sync with our routines, and us with theirs, that it seems almost like it was always so, and it can be hard to remember a time before that animal arrived. The termination stage can be like this; the behaviour is a normal and usual part of who you are or what you do. Often those I know who are in the termination stage find it difficult to even imagine that they did the previous behaviour. Those who no longer smoke, for example, may find it very difficult to even believe that they once did so. It can almost feel like it happened to someone else, not them.

12.3   Why Support People Who Are in the Maintenance Stage of Change?

When an owner has successfully made a change, it is easy for people around them such as workers, other professionals, colleagues, friends, and family to become complacent about the person's change. Others may believe that the owner will continue the behaviour change and no longer needs support, monitoring, help, or even anyone asking how they are doing. In this stage, like any of the other stages of change, slipping back into old behaviours is possible (3.9, 10.12). It is key, then, for owners to have continued offered support for their behaviour change and help to maintain it.

At the start of making a behaviour change, in the action phase (3.6), people can receive a good deal of positive reinforcement from others about their change. People will notice and often comment and tell the person how well they are doing. For the individual themselves, in the action stage, the reasons for changing are often clear in their minds and easy to remember. However, change, especially in the maintenance stage, can become a bit of a slog. It is easy to forget the reasons for making the change and the benefits it brings. Instead the old behaviour may come to mind with wistful thinking about it. People may start to imagine doing the behaviour again, believing it could be done just once or twice as they have the change cracked and everything under control. This can often be the slippery slope back to the old behaviour. Added to this is the likely reduction or loss of reinforcement and acknowledgement from others. Think back to a behaviour you have changed in the past, perhaps something like stopping smoking, reducing alcohol, or eating a healthy diet. You may remember how, after a period of making the change, it became easy to think about the old behaviour with increasing affection. It is possible to fool ourselves that 'just the one' (cigarette, glass of wine on a day we have planned not to drink, or an unhealthy treat to eat) wouldn't matter and that we have got this thing under control.

Prochaska and DiClemente highlighted that most people don't make a sustained behaviour change the first time around, and many have to have a number of attempts before they are successful (3.9). They say that those undertaking change need support to help them learn from the times that were not successful.

There is a risk that without this help, people can just continue with a trial-and-error approach to change, which often doesn't result in a sustained change. If this trial-and-error approach does eventually work, it has taken a lot of time, effort and energy. The alternative could have been a change successfully undertaken and maintained earlier, with some helpful learning from the lapses or relapses or slips and trips (10.12).

So, how can we help people who are making changes to succeed and maintain their changes?

The first, perhaps, is to be prepared to invest, for the long haul, in owners when they are making change. It is easy to view the continuation of support, when a change has been made, as costly and not needed. However, with what we now know about the stages of change and the likelihood of lapses or relapses, slips and trips in behaviour change, we can perhaps see that *not* supporting owners can create more work for us, or others, in the future, and can have an impact on the health and welfare of their animals.

If people keep returning to see workers, or workers have to continue to visit in welfare cases because required changes have not been made, it can be disheartening for owners and workers alike. When this happens, it can change the relationships workers have with owners. Owners may dread seeing workers or stop engaging with individuals, organisations, or anyone at all.

Workers can feel frustrated, angry, and believe that owners have wasted their time and not taken advice. Experiences like this can lead to burnout for some workers.

If we can view lapses in behaviour change as a common and normal part of what happens in behaviour change (3.9) and that people need support at all the stages of the change, not just at the start, we can make a real difference to them, their animals, and also to our own experiences of our work.

12.4   How We Might Support People in the Maintenance Stage

We can support people in the maintenance stage by, first, offering them follow up. It doesn't have to be that often or time consuming. Meeting in person or by phone or on a remote or online platform can allow us to review their progress and experiences. When workers do this in a structured way, owners can be supported to make meaningful change. They can identify what has worked and not worked for them and then apply this learning, as opposed to going through the exhausting yo-yoing trial and error approach.

At the maintenance stage, owners often have a wealth of experience from making the change or changes. They now have their own expertise (4.7.2) of the change process for their issues. All that may be required is brief help to reflect and review what is successful for them and what may need to be adapted slightly, or if their situation changes or life events occur, how they maintain the change alongside these. There is a lovely French word, *bricoler,* which can mean to tinker, adapt, potter. At this stage in making a change, people often need to tinker, make slight alterations and adjustments to how they are implementing change. Workers can help owners to review their progress and experiences and bricoler or tinker with their goals and plans (10.4–10.10).

We can ask owners to report the progress of change and the following questions can be of use:

- What are your concerns about the future?
- What concerns do you have about what might get in the way of you sustaining the change?
- What are the situations / thoughts / feelings in which you are most likely to slip back or are most likely to trip you up?
- What do you think is the best way to cope with those situations?
- What has worked before or recently?
- What might work again and what would you not bother trying in future?
- What do you think we need to do? How can I help? How can others help?
- What kind of support do you think you need?
- What else do we need to do?
- How realistic is your plan?

Box 12.3   Exercise

If you have started to use the ideas, philosophy, structures and techniques outlined in this book to make some changes to how you work, ask yourself the maintenance questions above about how you will continue to work with behaviour change. Perhaps jot the answers down.
  What do you make of that?

As people move into action (3.6) and then the maintenance stage (3.7), they become very capable of dealing with the day-to-day issues that might trip them up or cause a slip. These, when repeated or experienced often, lead to the creation of habitual management or coping strategies. In the maintenance stage, confidence builds through the experience of actually performing the behaviour required for the change. This builds self-efficacy (11.15, 12.6). By now, owners are probably able to manage difficulties and moderate issues that occur from time to time and will have the capacity and ability to circumnavigate them.

However, in the maintenance stage, be aware of situations or experiences that happen rarely or infrequently. It is the unusual, unexpected, or infrequent issue that can now throw the change off track. These can be for a number of reasons as follows:

- Physical: This could be the owner experiencing an injury, pain or contracting a virus. Example: An owner who was doing well with managing their animals has a sudden knee injury, appendicitis, stroke or flu.
- Emotional: This could be something that causes happiness or sadness or another emotion such as despondency, hopelessness, anger, or anxiety. Example: This could be a wedding, a bereavement, divorce or the birth of a child. It could be an anniversary or a seasonal celebration such as Christmas or a holiday.
- Cognitive: This is when the owner's thinking is skewed towards having negative thoughts about themselves, their situation, or others. Example: This could be when they experience a loss of self-esteem (11.14) or return to an old pattern of thinking, experience poor mental health due to life difficulties or a mental illness such as depression.
- Situational: This may happen when they come across a physical place that is associated with old behaviour. Example: My friend and colleague Keith believed himself to be in the termination stage of a significant change. He had successfully stopped smoking for some years. That was until he went to France on holiday. He was at a particular Parisian café that he loved, having a drink in the sunshine with his wife, feeling that this was as good as life could get. Then he had the thought, 'What would make this even better? I know - a cigarette!' and so he started smoking again right there. This happened to Keith not once but twice. He twice started smoking again at that particular café in Paris.
- Interpersonal: This is often about conflict with others. Example: This could be feeling let down by others, ostracised, lonely, left out or having disputes with neighbours, someone on an equine yard, or authorities, or at work.

12.5   Supporting People to Develop Skills to Make Behaviour Changes

As consistently highlighted throughout this book, change is difficult, for all of us. People need skills to be successful in making behaviour changes. Self-efficacy (11.15 and 12.6 below) is essential, not only to starting to make a change but also for continuing it, making it stick in the maintenance stage and beyond.

An activity self-monitoring form can be found in Chapter 14 which may be of use to some owners to help them build reminders of what they have achieved.

12.6   Return to Self-efficacy

We all need skills to start, plan for, implement and to continue to make successful behaviour changes. Our self-efficacy, our belief in our ability to make a change, will wax and wane as we make the change. Bandura (1982) said, 'If self-efficacy is lacking, people tend to behave ineffectually, even though they know what to do'.

Self-efficacy is like the fuel in a car. Without fuel, a car won't go, may not even start out on a journey. A driver could possibly roll the car down a hill, an easy solution in the short term, but as soon as an incline or a difficulty is met, the vehicle will stop or even roll backwards.

People need skills to succeed with making changes. These skills may be ones that they need to develop or ones that are from the past, dormant, and need to be reawakened, brushed off, and put into use again. Sometimes, completely new skills need to be developed. People need support to make changes, but this does not always have to be time consuming or even that formal. Regular, small, steady drip-drip support from the right person, or persons, can be essential for the individual to support change and success.

12.7   Early Warning Signs

Finally, we might help owners to identify the early signs that they may be slipping back or are having difficulty in maintaining their behaviour change. Looking back, reviewing their experiences, perhaps by revisiting a timeline (7.3) for the behaviour, can help owners identify small but significant indicators that have started difficulties for them in the past. They might like to add these to their contingency plans (10.10). This means that we can discontinue our contact with them if it is no longer required, but they can return quickly and early to us or someone like us, should they identify an early warning sign.

12.8   Conclusion

This chapter considered the last stage of change, maintenance, and the possible further, final stage, termination, identified by Prochaska and DiClemente. A key message in this chapter has been that people still need some support and contact from workers even when it appears they have, for some time, been successful with a behaviour change. This support doesn't need to be that often or to take much time. It doesn't necessarily need to come from animal health, care, or welfare workers. Other people may be able to provide this support for an owner. What is important is that encouragement and help is factored into an owner's plan in ways that are meaningful for the individual.

References

Bandura, A. (1982) Self-efficacy Mechanism in Human Agency. *American Psychologist.* 37, 2, 122–147. ISSN 0003-066X. https://doi.org/10.1037/0003-066X. 37.2.122 (p. 127).

Prochaska, J. and Prochaska J. (2016) *Changing to Thrive.* Minnesota: Hazelden.

13

Looking Forward

13.1 Introduction

This is the last real chapter of the book – although Chapter 14, which follows, has templates and examples to support your work.

Throughout, this book is a challenge because readers are required to make changes in themselves in order to try, use and adopt the ideas and ways of working that it suggests. It needs alterations and amendments to the ways in which we approach people and the work undertaken with them. We may desperately want owners to make changes, for their own welfare as well as for that of their animals, and sometimes for their family members, communities and others affected by the situation and even the environment. However, to really help people, we need to be flexible and manage our drive to tell and fix people and their behaviours; we will need to fight the fixing reflex (2.2.8) and reduce or avoid using the traditional methods described in Chapter 2.

We all know that change is hard. For anyone. Hopefully the ideas, structures for conversations and techniques discussed in the preceding chapters have made sense, are appealing and you have started to use some, to test them out for yourself. You may be setting off to use these ideas with great gusto and enthusiasm. However, consider how you will get support or what else you need to ensure success. It is easy to find ideas, such as those contained in this book, appealing only for them to then be semi-forgotten under workloads that are often urgent, demanding and heavy.

13.2   How Behaviour Change and Motivational Interviewing (MI) Sits in Our Increasingly Complex World

It is becoming increasingly recognised that human, animal and environmental health are interconnected. Professionals and agencies from all of these areas should be finding ways to collaborate, and this is an emerging area known as the 'One Health' approach. Whilst the ideas in this book are from the human health field and well evidenced there, they transfer well into animal health. Human behaviour change, especially MI, should be central to One Health approaches.

The demands on animal health, care and welfare workers have perhaps never been so great. In the UK and other countries, companion ownership has increased, especially since the Covid-19 pandemic. There is a growth in the number of inexperienced and first-time animal owners. Alongside this is a rise in the demands and expectations upon vets and others, albeit with lesser understanding among owners about their part in good animal health care and welfare. The cost-of-living crisis arrived hot on the heels of the global pandemic and has brought new tensions and difficulties for both animal owners and workers. There is increased frustration among owners, often directed at workers, and even hostility and aggression.

Animal welfare organisations, charities and agencies have experienced increasing demands on their resources in recent decades, and there is no sign of any let up, especially in light of the increased levels of companion animal ownership and financial and practical difficulties for many. Breeding animals can be a lucrative income generator, and with increased demand comes increased levels of poor and indiscriminate breeding. Added to this, social media brings its own impact, enabling effortless and cost-free advertising of animals. It also provides a platform for unregistered, and at times unscrupulous, 'rescues' and 'sanctuaries' to establish their presence.

These complex and concerning issues are expected to persist, affecting workers regardless of their workplace or job roles. It is important to highlight that burnout among workers, stemming from employment conditions and heavy workloads, as well as compassion fatigue resulting from the emotional burden in animal health and welfare, are widely recognised.

Many things will be needed to support and sustain workers, but having increased ability and confidence in behaviour change conversations, often ones which are challenging and difficult, can be one of the factors that may help.

Those trained in MI and who continue to use and develop it within their work frequently report that it gives better outcomes with owners, including in complex and difficult cases. They also report that it helps them deal with challenging situations, including threatening or hostile people. Colleagues who use MI, in both human health and animal health and welfare, repeatedly report being happier in the work they do and taking less worries home with them. They experience a heightened sense of resilience, which enables them to better perform the highly demanding and often emotionally impactful work that is required of them.

13.3 Sustaining Momentum – Continuing to Use and Develop Skills in Using Behaviour Change Methods Including MI

Those who I have trained in MI and behaviour change over more than two decades tell me that the most important things they do to keep developing the skills are: consciously practicing the strategies and approaches (reflection-in-action); and continuously reviewing (reflection-on-action) (5.10) and returning to any elements or underpinning ideas they may not be using. Although I trained in MI, use it myself, taught it for over 20 years and now write about it, I too have to keep working at it. Writing this book has been part of that process for me, to keep developing and thinking about and using MI and the other ideas.

13.3.1 An Invitation to You

That is why, when I set out to write this book, I envisaged the reader returning to chapters and elements repeatedly, as needed, to allow learning to be built in layers. I invite you to not to leave this book on a shelf. Rather, I encourage you to take it out with you to clinics, on visits. Have it in your work vehicle, in your bag, on your desk – so that it is at hand, and you can dip in to it as a swift reminder of what might be used for a particular visit, client or owner. When I first started writing this book, in the first UK lockdown due to Covid-19, I always had a vision of this book being somewhat dog-eared, a little tatty and well-thumbed due to use. I hope this book becomes yours and is visibly well used. Feel free to add ideas and notes to it that will help you to integrate it into your work.

13.3.2 Ideas to Support Action and Maintenance in the Use of MI

Talk to other people about behaviour change, about MI, the other ideas in the book and your experiences. There are increasingly more people in the animal health and welfare world becoming interested in behaviour change and also in what MI can help us do. My colleagues and I are training people to use MI, so seek out like-minded people, possibly someone MI trained, and talk to them. Even consider attending a course or getting some support from someone MI trained, or accessing formal time to undertake reflection-on-action with another professional who can guide you with this. Get feedback on your conversations with others about change or possible change. Ask owners for feedback about how they found the conversation: often, this information about our work can be the most useful. After all, owners have some of the best expertise to tell us how we did and what worked.

Go back to the elements you find you *don't* use, or perhaps not regularly. For example, when I first trained, I initially avoided using the exploring ambivalence structure, the central core element for MI and behaviour change! As I am dyslexic, it seemed a bit too complicated. Now, as it should be, it is my main go-to in any conversation about change.

Remember that this book, like MI, is not designed to be followed in a regimented, linear way. Rather, it is designed and written for you, the reader, to revisit sections and chapters when needed and as judged by you. The book is like the conversations we have with people about change: there are rapid movements forwards and then a retracking back to reconsider thoughts, experiences, beliefs and ideas.

Have confidence in your skills. Don't think that all this stuff is new and it needs to be learnt anew, like a foreign language. You will, due to your work with animals and owners, already possess many of the skills and attributes needed. Your existing skills support these new ideas.

Chapter 10 looked at devising goals (10.4–10.6), action plans (10.9) and contingency plans (10.10), and contained an exercise that you were invited to complete. That exercise had a suggested pre-set goal for you of using MI and other ideas from this book in your practice. If you did that exercise, perhaps you could now revisit and review it. Make any changes that are needed with your experiences. If you didn't get to do the exercise then, perhaps you might like to do it now – you can find it replicated below. If you have been using the ideas and techniques for a while, you might like to ask yourself the questions from Chapter 12 (12.4) for maintenance stage, which you can also find below.

Many of those trained in MI tell us that it is useful for them to have visual reminders or prompts of what they might or could use in sessions. In the following chapter with templates and forms, you will find a diagram where, for each of the stages of change, MI and other strategies and ideas are listed. This may help you as a quick reminder or revision.

A new goal idea has been added to the exercise – *I will plan to use the following structures, techniques or ideas once a week in my work*. This invites you to identify which ideas or structures or techniques from this book you don't use or use less regularly, so that you can aim to use them more consistently. Some of the most common ones to forget are the exploring ambivalence (8.3), hypothetical look over the fence (9.3) and typical day (7.6). But, if you find you haven't used the timeline, the importance, confidence (and readiness) scales (7.11): or forget to spend time working on and agreeing the agenda (Chapter 6) with an owner, you might add these in. There may be the skills that can drop off our radar, such as reducing questions, especially closed questions (5.14), and using reflecting more often (5.16), aiming for a ratio of questions to reflecting two or even three reflective statements for every question used (see 5.14.2) and making any questions that are used open rather than closed (5.14.1.1). Hold in mind the need to hear and understand the owner's frame of reference (Chapter 1) or the backstory to their situation. Listening out for which stage of change (Chapter 3) the owner might be in right at that moment and adapting your stance and responses accordingly – perhaps dancing, not wrestling (4.10.1).

Box 13.1   Exercise

You might like to complete the action plan for the suggested goals below. With your experience so far, what might get in the way or trip you up for using these techniques and ideas? Then, consider contingency plans for these two goals and how you could mitigate what can trip you up.

Goal (suggested)	Action plan	Timescales	Who can help?
Using MI and other supporting ideas in my practice with animal owners to help them think about / make changes (this is a suggestion only, please amend to make it your goal)			
I will plan to use the following structures, techniques or ideas once a week in my work			

Goal	What might get in the way of your goal and action plan?	When? How?	Contingency plan
Using MI and other supporting ideas in my practice with animal owners to help them think about / make changes			
I will plan to use the following structures, techniques or ideas once a week in my work			

Questions we can ask owners to report the progress of change, and you might ask yourself these for your progress of using the ideas and strategies in this book.

- *What are your concerns about the future?*
- *What concerns do you have about what might get in the way of you sustaining the change?*
- *What are the situations / thoughts / feelings in which you are most likely to slip back, or which are most likely to trip you up?*
- *What do you think is the best way to cope with those situations?*
- *What has worked before or recently?*
- *What might work again, and what would you not bother trying again?*
- *Who can help? How can they help?*
- *What kind of support do you think you need?*
- *What else do you need to do?*
- *How realistic is your plan?*

13.4   Final Thoughts

Motivational Interviewing is not a bag of tricks to get people to do what we want them to. Success in these types of interventions is not so much due to the strategy or technique used: rather, it will be due to the worker, their approach and attitude and the skilled use of active listening.

Miller and Rollnick (2009) remind us that MI is not a panacea for all ills: rather, it is a strategy to use with people when they need to make changes. There will be times and places where it is not appropriate to use some, or any, of the ideas and techniques covered in this book. However, those who do integrate MI and the other behaviour change ideas successfully into their animal health and welfare work often find these can be used, in some way, in the majority of their practice.

Active listening is central to MI and any behaviour change work. Remember to undertake and practice quality listening in the same way a top athlete approaches their sport. It takes thought and practice but if all you do is listen, and do so really well, that alone with have a big impact on the work done and the results you get.

On one hand, be brave and focused in the conversations you have, and remember that working with people to make change is not just about being nice: it requires workers to take risks in their interactions and to help people discuss difficult and sometimes shameful issues. On the other hand, keep learning and be gentle with both your owners and yourself whilst maintaining a professional curiosity.

Thank you for reading this book. I hope you continue to use it and that the ideas within it serve you, and those you work with, well.

Reference

Miller WR, Rollnick S. 2009 Ten things that motivational interviewing is not. *Behavioural and Cognitive Psychotherapy.* 37(2):129–40. doi: 10.1017/ S1352465809005128. PMID: 19364414.

14

Templates and Appendices

14.1 Introduction

This chapter contains templates and an example to support you in your work. Each gives a link back to the chapter and section it relates to.

At the end, you will find a flow diagram. Those we teach often say they could do with something as an easy and quick reference guide to glance at prior to a visit or a consultation. This flow diagram is designed to be that quick-scan prompt or reminder. It is based on The Stages of Change Model and has suggested Motivational Interviewing (MI) strategies or other interventions mentioned in the book, which might be considered at each stage. There is also a third column that gives ideas of what types of approaches may be needed from us as workers.

14.2 Socratic Questioning (To Support Chapter 5, Section 5.14.3)

Adapted from R.W. Paul's six types of Socratic questions (Paul, R. and Elder, L. (2006). The Art of Socratic Questioning. Dillon Beach, CA: Foundation for Critical Thinking).

Below are some examples of questions we *could* use for Socratic questioning – however. remember that these need to be done in a non-interrogatory way: and when working with behaviour change, use reflections, mini summaries and summaries. You don't need to use them all, or in the order given. See the example questions below.

1. Use questions for clarification, such as:	What is it that we need to focus on? Can you say some more about that? What makes you see it/feel about it that way? What do you already know about the issue/situation/problem?
2. Questions that probe assumptions:	What evidence is there for this assumption/belief? And what evidence against? Is there anything we assume without having evidence? Could you explain why/how you arrived at that conclusion/ decision? What would happen if ...?
3. Questions that probe reasons and evidence:	What would be an example? Have you experienced something similar? Seen others do/ experience similar? What do you think causes _____ to happen? What experiences have you to support your answer/view?
4. Questions about viewpoints and perspectives:	What would someone else in a similar situation say? What would you say to someone in a similar situation? Is there an alternative view/explanation? What do you think causes other people to be concerned? What would be another way to look at it? What are the good things about _____? And what are the not-so-good things about _____? Have I got this right – that on the one hand, you think/feel _____, and on the other, _____.? How are _____ and _____ similar?
5. Questions that probe implications and consequences:	What are the consequences of _____? When you look ahead, what do you see if things don't change? And if they do change? How does changing or not changing affect you/others/your life? How does changing or not changing fit with your previous experiences? Why is this issue / change important?

14.3   Example of Socratic Questioning – Using a Guiding Style with Socratic Questioning to Help the Owner find the Answer Themselves (See 5.14.3)

This is an example of some Socratic questions used alongside reflections and mini summaries in a guiding style.

Scenario: Owner is struggling with their puppy and is considering giving it up/ rehoming it and buying a more 'suitable' one.

WORKER (W):   Tell me about what you're thinking right now around your puppy.

OWNER (O):   *Well, it's more daunting than I expected; I knew he would need a lot of attention, and there would be stuff I needed to do, but ...*

W: You expected some work and things for you to solve with a new puppy. What things had you expected?

O: *Well, that there would be the special food, I guess, and toilet training, and then how to train him to behave well and not bite people.*

W: You had expected all of those things, so what turned out to be different?

O: *I guess it was the whole scale of it, the time it has taken. I wasn't expecting that, and the sheer damage he does. We can't go on like this. And then the barking ... The neighbours have made complaints.*

W: You had foreseen some of the issues but not others such as the damage and complaints from others. You say you know you can't go on like this, and that something needs to change.

O: *Yeah, you know, we have thought seriously about handing the dog over to someone else and then finding a puppy that would be more suitable and less difficult.*

W: So, one option for you is to try again with another dog. What would be different?

O: *Well, I guess a smaller breed might be easier to handle, and a different dog would have a different temperament and not do these destructive things.*

W: The barking and chewing items are something only particular to your current dog.

O: *Well, no, I guess not when you put it like that. We had read all the books and stuff, and we knew there would be some difficult behaviours ...*

W: Just not this difficult, huh?

O: *Yeah, this seems extreme.*

W: Let me see if I have got where we are so far ... You really wanted this puppy and knew that puppies came with a need for lots of work in all sorts of ways from their owners, but you hadn't expected this much difficulty.

O: *Yes, that right. It's not been what we expected.*

W: What was it that you had expected?

O: *Well, we had envisaged a nice, happy puppy that would grow into a happy dog – which would be part of our family and we could do things with.*

W: And this hasn't happened.

O: *No, it's sad, isn't it, that things haven't turned out as we wanted? We didn't get the dog we wanted.*

W: You didn't get the dog that you wanted – it was the wrong dog for you?

O: *Yes, bless him, don't get me wrong – he has his lovely moments and he's really a nice dog underneath – but it's his behaviour, or some of it, that is just not right for us.*

W: Is there any other way of looking at this dog's behaviour, or thinking about it?

(Long pause)

O: *Well ... You know I have wondered if another dog, another puppy might be just the same or even worse!*

W: Can you say a bit more about that?

O: *Well, if we had another puppy, it would be all of that early work all over again – the toilet training and stuff. You know, with the current dog, at least we have done a lot of that.*

W: If you started again with another puppy, there would be work to do all over again, and it might be difficult to guarantee to not have similar behavioural issues as now.

O: *Yes! What if that happens?*

W: And, say you did get another puppy, and that did happen again ... What might that tell you?

(Long pause again)

O: *That ... it was us ... not the dog ... that we need to do something differently, and not expect the dog to.*

W: How might you test that idea out to see if it was true?

O: *I guess we could ask for help with our current dog to see if there was something we could do differently.*

W: Who might you ask?

O: *Well, there are dog trainers and experts and classes and stuff.*

W: Tell me some more about that ... What you know ...

14.4   Chapter 6, Section 13: Agenda Template (Adapted from Miller and Rollnick 2013)

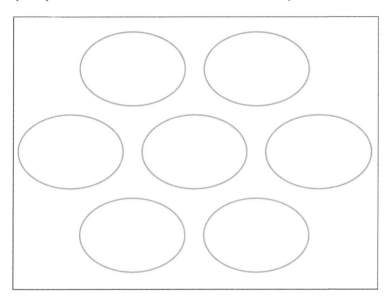

14.5   Chapter 7, Section 7.11: Importance, Confidence and Readiness Scales (Reference: Miller and Rollnick 2013)

Importance

← *not important*   *very important* →

0	1	2	3	4	5	6	7	8	9	10

Confidence

← *not confident*   *very confident* →

0	1	2	3	4	5	6	7	8	9	10

Readiness

← *not ready*   *very ready* →

0	1	2	3	4	5	6	7	8	9	10

14.6   Chapter 8, Section 3: Exploring Ambivalence Template (Adapted from Miller and Rollnick 2013)

Current behaviour _____	
The good things about _____	The not so good things about _____
Possible new behaviour/changed behaviour _____	
The not so good things about _____	The good things about _____

14.7   Chapter 11: Goals and Contingency Plans

Goals and Action Planning Template

Goal	Action plan	Timescales	Who can help?

14.8   Chapter 11: Contingency Planning Template

Goal	What might get in the way of your goal and action plan?	When? How?	Contingency plan

14.9 Chapter 11: Task/Activity Recording Sheet

Day → Activity/task ↓	.......day	.......day	.......day	.......day	.......day	.......day	.......day
Notes							

14.10 Chapter 11: Task Tick List

Day ____

Time	Task	Completed √	Notes

14.11 See Chapter 11 Box 11.11 for Information about How to Use This Self-Efficacy Scale for Yourself

Schwarzer, R., & Jerusalem, M. (1995). Generalized Self-Efficacy scale. In J. Weinman, S. Wright, & M. Johnston, Measures in health psychology: A user's portfolio. Causal and control beliefs (pp. 35-37). Windsor, UK: NFER-NELSON.

	Not at all true	Hardly true	Moderately true	Exactly true
I can always manage to solve difficult problems if I try hard enough.	☐	☐	☐	☐
If someone opposes me, I can find the means and ways to get what I want.	☐	☐	☐	☐
It is easy for me to stick to my aims and accomplish my goals.	☐	☐	☐	☐
I am confident that I could deal efficiently with unexpected events.	☐	☐	☐	☐
Thanks to my resourcefulness, I know how to handle unforeseen situations.	☐	☐	☐	☐
I can solve most problems if I invest the necessary effort.	☐	☐	☐	☐
I can remain calm when facing difficulties because I can rely on my coping abilities.	☐	☐	☐	☐
When I am confronted with a problem, I can usually find several solutions.	☐	☐	☐	☐
If I am in trouble, I can usually think of a solution.	☐	☐	☐	☐
I can usually handle whatever comes my way.	☐	☐	☐	☐

14.12 Chapter 12: Maintenance

Activity Self-Monitoring

What activities/tasks would you like to do/achieve in the next few days or week?	When you have achieved each, note down here what you notice about how you feel, what your thoughts are.	Note down any feedback or comments from others.

14.13   Stages of Change and MI Strategies

This diagram uses the stages of change and, for each stage, suggests MI strategies or other interventions mentioned in the book which might be considered at this stage. There is also a third column that gives guidance about what may be required from us as workers.

Stage of change	MI strategy/intervention	Required behaviour/attitude from worker
Pre-contemplation	• Gain and build <u>Rapport</u> • Watch for and reduce <u>Discord</u> • <u>Engagement</u> • Listen for stages of change • <u>Agenda</u> (multiple to single) • Revisit <u>Importance, Confidence</u> (and possibly <u>Readiness</u>) • <u>Typical day</u> • <u>Timeline</u> – looking back	• *Active listening* • *Open questions v Reflections* • *Be neutral!* • *Be curious* • *Be empathic* • *Be aware of your own agenda* • *Adapt approach to stages of change being indicated* • *Dancing not wrestling* • *Be collaborative* • *Think about follow or guide or direct* • *Watch for premature focus* • *Think process not outcome* • *Try and find out the 'backstory'* • *Relax into the work* • *Watch for the fixing reflex* • *Roll with Discord* • *Come back alongside the person (lead off the shoulder)*

Stage of change	MI strategy/intervention	Required behaviour/attitude from worker
Contemplation	• Recheck <u>Agenda</u> • Revisit <u>Importance, Confidence</u> (and possibly <u>Readiness</u>) • <u>Typical day</u> • <u>Explore Ambivalence</u> (the good and not so good) • <u>Timeline</u> – Looking back • <u>Hypothetical look over the fence</u> – Looking forward • <u>Beliefs and concerns</u> about change	• *Be neutral!* • *Be curious* • *Be aware of your own agenda* • *Be collaborative* • *Think about follow or guide or direct* • *Watch for premature focus* • *Think process not outcome* • *Relax into the work* • *Watch for the fixing reflex* • *Allow the person to be uncomfortable with the ambivalence* • *Don't make it ok or try to stop them being upset*

Stage of change	MI strategy/intervention	Required behaviour/attitude from worker
Preparation	• Recheck <u>Agenda</u> • Sort/address the practical issues • Revisit <u>Importance, Confidence</u> (and possibly <u>Readiness</u>) • Do or Revisit <u>Typical day</u> • Do or Revisit <u>Timeline</u> – Looking back • <u>Explore Ambivalence</u> (the good and not so good) • <u>Hypothetical look over the fence</u> – Looking forward • What might trip them up, and how would they manage this? • <u>Beliefs and concerns</u> about change • Support self-efficacy • Encourage them to explore other things/times when they have been successful, no matter how small or brief – a timeline might be useful	• *Be neutral!* • *Be curious* • *Be aware of your own agenda* • *Be collaborative* • *Think about follow or guide or direct – if they ask for information or direction, give information that they ask for – ask-offer-ask* • *Watch for premature focus* • *Think process not outcome* • *Relax into the work* • *Watch for the fixing reflex* • *Allow the person to be uncomfortable with the ambivalence* • *Don't make it ok or try to stop them being upset* • *Don't underestimate ambivalence!*

• Help develop self-esteem if needed • Think about others who have achieved change – modelling • Any groups/courses, etc., that they can use/attend? • Recording of behaviour if suitable for individual • Give tailored information – ask-offer-ask • Recording of behaviour if suitable for individual • Support problem-solving • Move towards <u>goal setting</u> – SMART and small at first • Draw up contingency plan	• *Don't be disheartened if they slip back one or more stages – adapt and come alongside them*

Stage of change	MI strategy/intervention	Required behaviour/ attitude from worker
Action	• Recheck <u>Agenda</u>, reset agenda if it has changed • Revisit <u>Importance, Confidence</u> (and possibly <u>Readiness</u>) • <u>Goal setting</u> – SMART and small at first • Review progress • Maybe revisit <u>Timeline</u> and add to it • Review what worked and what was difficult • Revisit <u>contingency plan</u> with this new experience/knowledge • Reset <u>goals</u> with new knowledge and experience • Recording of behaviour if suitable for individual • Recording of new behaviours if suitable for individual • Support self-efficacy • Support and encouragement	• *Be neutral!* • *Be curious* • *Be aware of your own agenda* • *Be collaborative* • *Think about follow or guide or direct* • *Think process not outcome – allow the person to fall into a hole and learn from it with support* • *Relax into the work* • *Watch for the fixing reflex* • *Don't underestimate ambivalence!* • *Don't be disheartened if they slip back one or more stages – adapt and come alongside them*

Stage of change	MI strategy/intervention	Required behaviour/attitude from worker
Maintenance	• Recheck <u>Agenda</u>, reset agenda if it has changed • Revisit <u>Importance, Confidence</u> (and possibly <u>Readiness</u>) • Review progress • Review what worked and what was difficult • Revisit <u>contingency plan</u> with this new experience/knowledge • Recording of new behaviours if suitable for individual • Support and encouragement – identify who can do this and how • Support self-efficacy	• *Be neutral!* • *Be curious* • *Be aware of your own agenda* • *Be collaborative* • *Think about follow or guide or direct* • *Think process not outcome – allow the person to fall into a hole and learn from it with support* • *Relax into the work* • *Watch for the fixing reflex* • *Don't underestimate ambivalence!* • *Don't be disheartened if they slip back one or more stages – adapt and come alongside them* • *Continue to offer support*

Miller, W. and Rollnick, S. (2013) *Motivational Interviewing: Helping People Change.* 3rd Ed. New York: Guilford Press.

Index

Practical Human Behaviour Change for the Health and Welfare of Animals,
First Edition. Bronwen Williams.
© 2024 John Wiley & Sons Ltd. Published 2024 by John Wiley & Sons Ltd.
Companion website: www.wiley.com/go/williams/human

Printed and bound by CPI Group (UK) Ltd, Croydon, CR0 4YY

29/08/2024

14547657-0001